You Are the ER Doc!

TRUE-TO-LIFE CASES FOR YOU TO TREAT

BY

PETER MEYER, MD

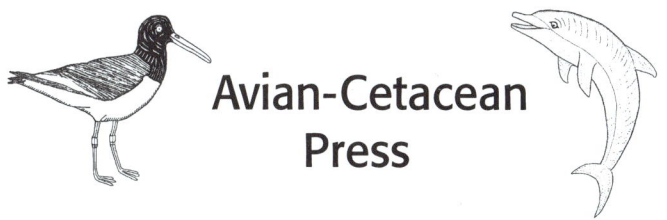

Avian-Cetacean Press

Copyright © 2001 by Peter Meyer

All rights reserved. No part of this book may be reproduced without written permission from the publisher or author, except by a reviewer, who may quote brief passages; nor may any part of this book be reproduced, stored in a retrieval system or transmitted in any form or by any other means, electronic, mechanical, photocopying, recording, or other, without written permission from the publisher or author.

Published by Avian-Cetacean Press in Wilmington, NC.
Printed and bound in the United States of America.

Cover photo by Catherine E. Meyer
Cover design by Wordwright Communications

Printing: 1 2 3 4 5 6 7 8 9 10

Comments and suggestions are welcome. Send communications to the author, c/o Avian-Cetacean Press, PO Box 15643, Wilmington, NC 28408.

Library of Congress Card Number: 00-108695

Publisher's Cataloging-in-Publication Data
Meyer, Peter, 1952—
   You Are the ER Doc! : True-to-Life Cases for You to Treat/ by Peter Meyer
p. 160
Includes index
ISBN: 0-9628186-2-3
1. Emergency medicine—Popular works 2. Hospitals—Emergency service—Popular works I. Title
RC87.M49 2001
616.02'5   00-108695
                                                                                CIP

Dedication

You Are the ER Doc! is dedicated to emergency medicine doctors in the trenches, those dedicated men and women who staff emergency departments day and night, weekday and weekend, regular day and holiday, 24 hours a day, 365 days a year.

You Are the ER Doc! is also dedicated to the emergency medicine nurses, technicians, clerks, and students, those dedicated men and women who co-staff emergency departments day and night, weekday and weekend, regular day and holiday, 24 hours a day, 365 days a year.

As the doctors, nurses, technicians, clerks, and students know, often the only thanks they get is the satisfaction of a job done well.

Disclaimer

You Are the ER Doc! is one doctor's opinion on the practice of emergency medicine and patient care. *You Are the ER Doc!* is not a rigid textbook, an ultimate treatise on the practice of emergency medicine, or the only way to practice medicine and care for patients. As in any profession (medicine, too!), problems can be solved in many different ways. The solutions to the patients' problems presented in this book are simply one doctor's concepts of patient care.

The patients described in *You Are the ER Doc!* do not represent individual patients treated by the author. Instead, they represent a compendium of the thousands of patients treated by the author during his emergency medicine career. The author, Peter Meyer, MD, endeavored to make as certain as possible that the names of patients in the book are fictitious, that they do not represent the names of actual patients treated by him. If the patients described match real persons in name and/or description, the resemblance is entirely coincidental.

Introduction

Emergency doctors care for all patients who enter the doors of the emergency department. Patients range from homeless alcoholics to notable members of society's upper crust. Ages range from newborn to centenarian (100 or over). The emergency doctor must be adept at treating all patients, be they poor or rich, young or old, sick or just worried, sane or mentally unstable.

The illnesses of patients presenting for emergency care range from simple to extremely complex. One patient may need a splinter removed from a finger; the next patient may be in total body failure. One patient may just need a doctor's excuse to miss work; the next might need to be yanked back out of death's door.

An emergency doctor never knows what will walk, roll, or be dragged through the doors of the emergency department; this uncertainty is both one of the tensions and one of the pleasurable challenges of practicing emergency medicine.

Emergency doctors should stand proud: Patient care is their top priority. Emergency doctors do not ask for payment before they embark on treating any patient in serious need.

Emergency departments have evolved into the "safety net" for patients in the United States. If a patient has no place else to turn, emergency department doors are always open. The Hippocratic tradition of honoring the patient-doctor relationship is alive and well in the "ER." May it so remain.

How to Use this Book

You Are the ER Doc! is meant to be enjoyable and entertaining. The stories can be read silently by individual readers, or the stories can be read aloud to one another.

You Are the ER Doc! is also designed to educate readers about emergency medicine, medicine in general, and human health.

Each story can be read in minutes. No particular sequence needs to be followed.

The situations described require active thought on the part of the reader. The reader may not always agree with the "correct" answer provided in the text. This difference of opinion does not make the author or the reader right or wrong.

The goal of *You Are the ER Doc!* is to promote interest and logical reasoning in medical matters. The author believes that modest medical knowledge, a practical approach, and a modicum of common sense can go a long way toward optimal patient care. See if you agree.

Contents

Magic Awakening	9
Low Belly Pain, Low Blood Pressure	12
Jehovah's Jeopardy	15
Bare-Butt Operation	18
Perfect Passing	22
Fever and Headache	27
Religious Refusal	30
Bleach Boy	33
Bugged	37
Taillight Sign	42
Squirrel Bite	45
Fox Lick	48
Granny's Pain	51
Handy Dandy	54
Fever in a Four Year-Old	58
A Baby with Fever	61
Moped Malady	64
Reptile GI Blues	68
Seizure	72
BB Boo-Boo	76
Bean in the Nose	79
Bladder Ballast	82

Chest Pain	85
Chest Pain/HMO	88
Big Bart	92
Wormy Meal	99
To Tube, or not to Tube	102
Pulling the Plug	105
Surprise Package	109
The Alcoholic	115
Belly Buster	118
Intubation Practice	122
Brave with Knives, Scared of Needles	125
Hip Fracture?	129
Bitten in Person	132
Tricky Trauma	135
Get the Lead Out?	138
The Drip	142
The Pregnancy Pukes	146
Snakebit	152
Snakebite	155
Index	158
Order Form	160

*No man is more worthy of esteem than
a physician who exercises his art
with caution and gives equal attention
to the rich and the poor.*

— Voltaire (1694 - 1778)

Magic Awakening

You are the emergency medicine doctor on duty in the Hometown Hospital Emergency Department. The time is midnight.

"I brought you some coffee."

Nurse Able hands you a cup of steaming, black java.

"Thanks, Able. I need it tonight. As cold as it is outside, I don't think we'll be busy. Of course, I don't want to hex us by predicting a quiet night."

Almost on cue, the emergency department radio sounds off.

"Medic-10 to Hometown Hospital."

Able rolls her eyes. "You did it. We're doomed!"

"Sorry."

Your finger presses the red talk button on the radio.

"Go ahead, Medic-10."

"We have a 24-year-old male, probable heroin overdose. He's not breathing. We're bag-breathing him. Can't get an IV line in. We're two minutes out."

"Critical set up," you order, striding toward Treatment Room 1.

The nurses are already ahead of you, darting into the room.

You don a blue gown, protective goggles and gloves, then pause to take a deep breath and gather your wits.

The ambulance glides to a halt outside the glass doors of the emergency department. The vehicle's flashing red lights create a strobe-like effect on the white walls inside.

Three green-uniformed paramedics spill out of the ambulance and initiate a Chinese fire drill-like protocol: Around to the back of the vehicle they dash. A stretcher is wrenched from the back of the ambulance. Paramedics, patient, and gurney roll

YOU ARE THE ER DOC!

into the emergency department as one, the paramedics continuing to work on the patient until they deliver their charge to you.

On the stretcher is a thin, white male, clothed in a pair of gray sweat pants, bare from the waist up. He lies still, lifeless. His skin color, at least, is pink — the oxygen forced into his lungs by the paramedics is working.

Your fingers probe the patient's neck.

"Strong carotid," you declare. "Where'd you find him?"

"In the bathroom of a downtown bar," one paramedic answers.

The paramedic holds out his hand, palm up. "We found this syringe next to his body. His friend said he was shooting heroin."

Question 1 — You should:
- A) Not touch the patient since he is high-risk for AIDS.
- B) Tell the paramedics to bag-breathe the patient several hours, until he wakes up.
- C) Put a breathing tube into the patient to breathe for him.
- D) Call a priest to give the patient his last rites before stopping the bag-breathing.
- E) Put in an IV line so you can give magic medicine.

Answer —
E) is correct.

"Got to have an IV!" you say. "Able, you take one arm, I'll take the other."

Your fingers wrap a tourniquet around the patient's right upper arm. You scan his elbow crease and forearm, looking for purple veins. Rows of tiny scabs and bruises on his limb offer mute testimony to intravenous drug use.

"A road map of needle marks," you state.

Your gloved fingertip slides over the rows of scabs, feeling hard, gnarly bumps — not soft, pliable veins.

"Damn," you swear softly.

Nurse Able snaps her tourniquet off the left arm.

"Nothing here," she says. "He's blown all his veins by shooting up."

Question 2 — You should:

A) Say a quick prayer, asking for help in finding a vein.
B) Stick a breathing tube into the patient's trachea so medicine can be given into his lungs through the tube.
C) Stick a big needle into the patient's tibia (lower leg bone) so medicine can be given into his bone marrow.
D) Stick a big needle into the patient's groin to find a deep vein.
E) Stick a needle into one of the patient's neck veins.

Answer —

All of the above are reasonable. You must get medicine into the patient, one way or another.

Moving up to the patient's head, you scan his neck. An earthworm-shaped bulge stands out on one side.

"My prayer has been answered," you say. "IV catheter, please."

A technician slaps the IV apparatus into your hand. Your left hand swipes over the patient's neck vein with an alcohol pad. Your right hand guides a needle through the patient's skin, into the purple worm-like line beneath. Red blood fills the syringe attached to the needle. With your index finger, you slide the plastic catheter off the needle into the vein.

"Tape it down, please," you say. "Give Sleeping Beauty here the Magic Kiss Medicine. Two milligrams of Narcan IV push. See if that doesn't wake him up and get him breathing."

Twenty seconds later, the young man sits bolt upright.

"Where am I?" he asks.

"At the Hometown Hospital Emergency Department," says Nurse Able.

"Just back from death's door," you add. "We yanked you back from the other side."

The young man lies back on the stretcher.

"Man, that was some good stuff," he says.

"Depends how you define good, doesn't it?" you counter.

He rolls over on his side.

"Get me a blanket," he says. "I'm cold." ❖

Low Belly Pain, Low Blood Pressure

Your next patient is: Anita Frankel, a 29 year-old female.

"Doctor, there's a lady in Room 8 that you need to see right away," Nurse Able reports. "She's hurting in her belly. Her blood pressure is low, 80 over 50."

"Let's go," you respond, striding toward Room 8 with the nurse at your side.

Mrs. Frankel lies on the stretcher with her eyes closed, her lips moving silently. Her arms curve and meet where her hands press on her lower abdomen.

Is she praying? you wonder.

"Mrs. Frankel, I'm the emergency doctor on duty. Can you tell me where you hurt?"

"Where my hands are, down low on the right side," she says.

Beads of sweat glisten on Mrs. Frankel's forehead. Her skin is pale and cool to touch. Instinctively, you circle her wrist with your fingers, searching for a pulse.

Fast and thready. Not good.

"When did your belly start to hurt?"

"A couple days ago. Maybe even a week. But all of a sudden tonight, it got real bad."

"Any fever or vomiting?"

"No."

"Diarrhea or blood in the stool?"

"No."

"Burning on urination? Frequency of urination?"

"No, I'm going just like normal."

"Discharge or bleeding from the vagina?"

"I've been spotting a little bit this week. I just thought my period was coming on late."

"When was your last period?"

"Six weeks ago. It was light then, too."

Question 1 — Possible causes of the patient's pain include:
A) Cyst on the ovary.
B) Appendicitis.
C) Kidney stone or infection.
D) Infection of the womb and fallopian tubes.
E) Ectopic pregnancy.
F) All of the above.

Answer —
F) is correct. *All* of the above are possibilities.

Question 2 — The most serious of these potential problems is:
A) Cyst on the ovary.
B) Appendicitis.
C) Kidney stone or infection.
D) Infection of the womb and fallopian tubes.
E) Ectopic pregnancy.

Answer —
E) is correct. Ectopic pregnancy, or pregnancy outside the womb, is the most serious potential diagnosis. A pregnancy in the fallopian tube can grow and eventually rupture the tube, causing hemorrhage (severe bleeding) inside the abdomen. A patient can bleed to death very quickly. The other conditions are potentially serious, but they do not require immediate treatment.

"It hurts every place you press," says Mrs. Frankel, as your hand pushes on her abdomen. She winces each time you apply pressure. Her abdomen feels tight.

"It hurts the most there." She scrunches her face as you press on her right lower abdomen.

"We need to send a pregnancy test," you tell Nurse Able, who is standing at the bedside.

"The triage nurse got a urine specimen and sent it as soon as Mrs. Frankel hit the door. The lab called the results just a minute ago."

She hands you a slip of yellow paper.

Thank God for my good emergency nurses.

"POSITIVE pregnancy test" reads the lab slip.

Your own pulse quickens.

Question 3 — You should:
  A) Start IV fluids.
  B) Monitor the patient's blood pressure closely; send blood tests for hemoglobin (blood level) and for type and crossmatch (for possible transfusion).
  C) Contact the patient's ob-gyn doctor.
  D) Notify the operating room of likely emergency surgery.
  E) All of the above.

Answer —
  E) is correct.

Without missing a beat, you spew orders at Nurse Able. "We need two IV lines. Run a liter of fluid in wide open. Check blood pressures every five minutes and let me know if there's a change. Notify the OR of imminent surgery and page Dr. Bradley stat."

"We've got a problem here," you tell Mrs. Frankel. "The pregnancy test is positive. You may have an ectopic pregnancy, outside the womb, in one of your fallopian tubes. You might be bleeding inside. I think you're going to need emergency surgery to find out and stop the bleeding if it is an ectopic."

A tear trickles down Mrs. Frankel's cheek.

"Doctor, can you get my husband back here and explain this to him, too?"

"Of course. We'll get him right away."

Good job, doctor. No indecision in this instance.
Most cases in the emergency department allow time to think the situation through. Some cases don't, and quick action is needed. Mrs. Frankel's predicament is a true emergency. ❖

JEHOVAH'S JEOPARDY

Your patient is: Anita Frankel, a 29 year-old female with abdominal pain and low blood pressure. She has asked you to explain your diagnosis and recommendation for surgery to her husband.

"Right in here, Mr. Frankel," a nurse says.

A tall, solidly-built man, with a handlebar mustache, strides into the room. He steps to his wife's side and grasps her hand in his. With his other hand, he pushes wisps of brown hair back from her forehead.

"You OK, honey?" he asks.

His wife's lower lip quivers, but she maintains control. "I'm still hurting," she says. "The doctor says I need surgery right away."

Mr. Frankel turns and looks you in the eye. "What's the situation, doctor?"

"Your wife has pain on one side of the lower abdomen. Her blood pressure is low. We ran a pregnancy test and it's positive. We have to assume she has an ectopic pregnancy, a pregnancy in her fallopian tube, until we know otherwise. She may be bleeding internally. She could bleed to death if we don't operate — soon."

"Has Dr. Bradley been in yet?"

"No, I've called her, and she's on the way."

"Can we wait to decide until after she sees my wife?"

"Yes and no. Dr. Bradley will look at your wife very quickly and then give her opinion, too. I am certain she'll agree with me and recommend immediate surgery. We need to make plans in that direction, at least. If Dr. Bradley feels otherwise, we can always hold our horses."

"We don't have any other choice, do we?" Mr. Frankel asks. "Not really."

Mr. Frankel squeezes his wife's hand in both of his. "Have you told him yet, about no blood products?"

Mrs. Frankel bites her lip and shakes her head no.

"We're Jehovah's Witnesses," Mr. Frankel says. "Under no circumstances is my wife to be given blood products of any type."

Question 1 — You should:
A) Contact the hospital's lawyer.
B) Contact the Frankels' lawyer.
C) Contact both lawyers and let them grope with the issue.
D) Tell Mr. Frankel his family's religious beliefs don't matter.
E) Make sure Mrs. Frankel's desire is as her husband states, and make sure she understands the implications.

Answer —
E) is correct. The patient must speak for herself. No one, not even her husband, can make this decision for her, if she is mentally competent to make her own decision.

"Mrs. Frankel, is what your husband says correct?"

"Yes," she says, with the slightest hesitation.

"There's a chance you could bleed to death, that you could die from loss of blood. Are you sure you want us to hold off on giving you blood if your life is at stake?"

Mrs. Frankel looks up at her husband. "Courage," he says.

"No blood, doctor," she states.

Question 2 — You should:
A) Stomp your feet and pull your hair.
B) Tell Mrs. Frankel to find another doctor, that you can't continue to treat her because her religious beliefs are different from yours.
C) Halt plans for any further treatment.
D) Order a blood transfusion to be given even if Mrs. Frankel refuses.
E) Comply with the patient's wishes and treat her to the best of your ability within the guidelines she sets forth.

Answer —
> E) is correct.

"Mrs. Frankel, you're an adult capable of making your own decisions. We will respect your beliefs and not give you blood products even under life-threatening circumstances. We'll do everything else we can to save your life."

Good care, doctor. Remember, your purpose is to help patients, not to fight them. As long as adult patients are mentally competent (not insane, brain-injured, under the influence of drugs or alcohol, etc.), they should be allowed to make decisions about their own treatment. ❖

Bare-Butt Operation

Your patient is: Candace Trent, a 15 year-old female with a bee sting.

"Hi, Ms. Trent, how are you?" you ask.

"Fine," the young lady answers.

She's a younger, carbon-copy of another woman in the room with her. They're both small in size, thin, with brown hair pulled back in a short ponytail.

"Ms. Trent's mother, I assume," you direct to the older version. "Or is it older sister?" you add, hedging your bet.

"Her mother is correct, but thank you, just the same," she answers. "I know Candace's problem is not a real emergency, but she got stung by a bee the other day, and the area just keeps getting bigger and redder. And the burning and itching kept her up almost all night last night."

"When were you stung?" you ask the young lady.

"Two days ago. It was just a regular honeybee."

"Any breathing difficulty or throat swelling?"

"No."

"Where did it sting you?"

Ms. Trent puts her head down. Her face flushes red.

"It got her on the behind," her mother offers. "She's embarrassed."

"Don't be embarrassed," you say. "Here in the emergency department, we see all kinds of private body parts every day and it doesn't mean anything to us."

"But it's not *your* butt," the young lady offers, smiling a little.

"No, it's not," you say, smiling yourself.

Question 1 — You should:
  A) Offer to check Ms. Trent alone, without anyone else in the room.
  B) Offer to check Ms. Trent with either her mother or any member of your staff in the room.
  C) Offer to check Ms. Trent with either her mother or a female member of your staff in the room.
  D) Suggest you video tape Ms. Trent's exam to show to a group of boy scouts you are instructing in first aid.
  E) Make a diagnosis and treatment without examining the patient.

Answer —
  C) is correct. Never put your patient, or yourself, in a situation allowing any question of sexual harassment.

"Ms. Trent, would you like your mother or one of my female staff members in the room when I take a look at the sting site?"

The young lady looks at her mother. "My mom, please," she answers.

Her mother nods reassuringly.

"OK, Ms. Trent," you direct. "Hop up on the table and lie down on your stomach."

The young lady complies. She lies face down, elbows propping her up, hiding her face in her hands.

You pull back Ms. Trent's gown, exposing the young lady's backside.

"Pretty good-sized reaction," you judge. On Ms. Trent's right buttock, extending up onto her back, is a fiery red, raised area, set off from the surrounding skin by sharp borders. A dark red dot, the size of a BB, marks the center of the red area.

Pulling a tape measure from your pocket, you stretch the tape over the red area, top-to-bottom first, then side-to-side.

"Twenty-one by sixteen inches," you say. "That's the largest local reaction to a bee sting that I've ever seen, I believe."

"Great," the young lady says. "A world record, on my butt, no less."

Question 2 — You should advise:

A) Applying cold packs to the red area as much as possible.
B) Taking Benadryl (diphenhydramine), an antihistamine available over-the-counter, four times a day.
C) Elevating the area as possible.
D) Checking for a stinger left in the sting site.
E) All of the above.

Answer —

E) is correct.

"Although this is an unusually large local reaction to a bee sting, the mainstay of treatment is simple: Rest the area, elevate the area, and apply cold — lots of cold, and take an antihistamine like Benadryl."

"So what you're telling me," Ms. Trent says, "is that I have to rest my butt, stick it up in the air, and freeze it off, all at the same time."

You smile. "Or we could go ahead and do a buttectomy, a behind removal."

"No, thanks!"

"One other thing I need to do is look closely with magnifying glasses, to check for a stinger left in the wound."

"Great. Now you're going to magnify my butt, as if it isn't big enough already."

"Be back in just a minute. Don't run off."

"I doubt I'm going to run out of here and flash everyone in the place," comes the reply.

You return to the room with magnifying glasses on. Sitting on a stool next to the stretcher, you direct a bright, overhead surgical light onto the young lady's backside.

Gently, you poke at the dark spot in the middle of the red area with your gloved finger.

"I take it this is where the bee stung you?"

"Right there at the bull's-eye. The bee flew right up my shorts. Lucky me."

With magnification, you spot a tiny, black, splinter-like object sticking up from the middle of the dark spot. Carefully, you grasp the object with a pair of tweezers and pull.

"Ouch!" says the young lady.

Holding the object close to your magnifying glasses, you view a miniature harpoon, barbed on the end.

"Eureka!" you say. "A stinger, still in the wound, continuing to release toxin and causing a bigger reaction. Now that the stinger is out, I believe you'll get better."

"Thank you, doctor," says Candace's mother. "And please excuse Candace's comments. She has a sharp tongue sometimes."

"No problem. I've rather enjoyed her banter. A sense of humor helps in coping with life's little calamities."

"Well, I'm glad you understand. I didn't mean to be a pain in the butt," the young lady adds.

"Understood," you respond. ❖

You Are the ER Doc!

Perfect Passing

You take a few sips of seltzer water, then set the plastic bottle on the desk. Spread in front of you is a patient's chart, the squares and boxes beckoning to be filled. The chart details the treatment of a three year-old boy, a screamer, whose head you just sewed up.

Paperwork, paperwork, you think. *Too much paperwork.*

The radio in the emergency department crackles to life.

"Medic-1 to Hometown Hospital."

Pushing the red talk button on the radio, you answer.

"Go ahead, Medic-1."

"We are enroute with a 75 year-old female we picked up at a church. She had the sudden onset of left arm numbness, then became poorly responsive. She's now unconscious, not responding to us at all. Her respirations were decreased, at 10 per minute, when we picked her up, but with oxygen they're up to 16, normal."

"Any history of diabetes?" you ask.

"No history of any medical problems," the paramedic continues. "We checked a blood sugar, it's normal at 105."

Question 1 — The most likely cause of the patient's problem is:
A) A heart attack.
B) Tick bite paralysis.
C) A whole-body infection.
D) Some kind of stroke.
E) A drug overdose, probably narcotics.

Answer —
D) is correct. The rapid appearance of an unconscious state suggests a problem with brain function. Narcotic drug overdose in a 75 year-old female at church is possible, but unlikely.

The green-uniformed paramedics lift the patient off the gurney and onto the hospital stretcher.

22

"What's her name?" you ask.

"Evita McKinney," one of the medics answers.

You put your face next to the patient's head.

"Mrs. McKinney," you say loudly. "Mrs. McKinney!"

Mrs. McKinney lies still, her eyes closed. She responds not a glimmer.

You pinch her upper arm between your index finger and thumb. No response. With a fisted hand, you rub her breastbone. No response.

"Not even responding to noxious stimuli," you state. "Vitals?" you ask.

"Blood pressure 200 over 90," Nurse Able answers. "Pulse 60, a little erratic. Respirations 16, erratic, too."

Mrs. McKinney's skin color is normal, pink. Her breathing pattern alternates every 30 seconds: deep breaths at a normal rate first, followed by shallow and slow breaths.

"Dim the lights a second, please," you ask. Lifting Mrs. McKinney's eyelids, you shine a penlight onto her black pupils. Both pupils are tiny, black dots. They do not constrict to the bright light.

"Did you give Narcan on the way in?" you ask a paramedic.

"We did. No response."

"Well, it's definitely not narcotics constricting her pupils, or the Narcan would have reversed it. She must have had a bleed into her brain, a massive stroke."

Nurse Worthy pulls back the blue curtain in the front of the room. "Doctor, there's a priest here from this lady's church. He says he needs to see you right away."

"OK. Let him come back."

Nurse Worthy ushers the young man into the room. He is clad in black pants and shirt, a clerical collar around his neck.

"I'm Father Franks," the young man introduces himself. "Thank you for letting me come back. Mrs. McKinney insisted if anything like this ever happened that I show you this."

Father Franks hands you a piece of paper.

"She carried this in her purse at all times."

The title at the top of the paper reads, *Declaration of Desire for a Natural Death*. The document is signed at the bottom by

You Are the ER Doc!

Mrs. McKinney and properly notarized.

"Mrs. McKinney was adamant," the priest says. "She wants extraordinary treatments withheld if her condition is terminal and incurable."

"We'll try to honor that request," you answer, returning the paper to the priest. "Tell me what happened to Mrs. McKinney."

"We were sitting around a table at our church, sorting food baskets for needy families. Mrs. McKinney was her usual happy self, telling us about a recent trip to Disney World with her grandchildren. Then, all of a sudden, she said her left hand and arm felt numb. No more than a couple minutes later, her eyes clouded over and her head slumped onto the table."

Question 2 — You should:
A) Order a stat CAT scan of the brain.
B) Order a blood count and urine drug screen.
C) Call Dr. Kevorkian.
D) Stop the oxygen and IV fluids.
E) Send Mrs. McKinney home to die.

Answer —
A) is correct. You must know what is causing Mrs. McKinney's symptoms. A CAT scan will show you if she has had a bleed into her brain.

"Call radiology, please, Able. Order a stat CAT scan of the brain. We've got to find out if Mrs. McKinney's ruptured a blood vessel in her brain."

"Her breathing is a bit more erratic," Able says. "After what her priest said, what should we do if her breathing stops?"

Question 3 — You should:
A) Tell Nurse Able to have the priest administer last rights.
B) Let the priest go with Mrs. McKinney to the X-ray department.
C) Call the lawyer who drafted Mrs. McKinney's *Declaration of Desire for a Natural Death* document. Ask for an exact definition of "extraordinary measures."
D) Tell Nurse Able to bag-breathe Mrs. McKinney and prepare to put a tube in Mrs. McKinney's trachea.
E) Let the priest decide what treatment Mrs. McKinney should get.

Answer—
   D) is correct.

"If she stops breathing, bag her and call me stat. I'll run over and intubate her. We can put her on a respirator until we get the CAT scan done. Right now, we don't know for sure what Mrs. McKinney's problem is."

"All right. We're off to CAT scan. I'll ask the X-ray tech to bring you the films as soon as they're ready."

Twenty minutes later, the tech hands you an X-ray folder. You slide the celluloid films into place on the X-ray viewboxes.

One look at the films gives the answer. The oval skull shows up light, the brain substance inside dark and speckled. In the midst of the dark pattern is an irregular, splotchy, white shape.

Nurse Able tugs on your sleeve. "I just brought Mrs. McKinney back. Her breathing is really slowing down. What do you want to do?"

"Here's the problem." You put your index finger on the white area on the film. "A big bleed. There's really no hope for functional recovery with a bleed this size."

   Question 4—You should:
   A) Call the priest back in to administer last rights.
   B) Send Mrs. McKinney home.
   C) Get the defibrillator warmed up in case Mrs. McKinney's heart stops.
   D) Put a tube in Mrs. McKinney's trachea and put her on the respirator.
   E) Stop the oxygen and take out the IV line.

Answer—
   A) is correct.

Nurse Able and you walk out of the room.
"If you have to go, that's the way to die," you remark.
"What do you mean?" Able asks.
"If anyone has a chance to make it past the Pearly Gates into Heaven, it's Mrs. McKinney. Think about it. She's doing volunteer work for the needy at her church when the stroke hits. She's got "no-code" papers in her pocketbook, which her priest delivers

to us promptly. We get the diagnosis quickly, so we don't tube her and keep her alive on the respirator. And the priest is right here to administer last rights."

"Yeah, I see what you mean. Kind of the perfect death, isn't it?"

"Yes, indeed. The perfect death. We should all be so lucky."

Medical note: Planning is important to facilitate death with dignity. Careful discussion with family members prior to medical debility is essential. Legal documents, such as a living will and a health care power of attorney, also help insure a person's wishes for end-of-life care are fulfilled. ❖

Fever and Headache

Your patient is: Abraham Alms, a 6 year-old with fever.

Your ten-hour shift is nearly over. You sit in a cubicle, your head bent over the mass of paperwork involved in caring for patients.

Your record-keeping reverie is broken by the presence of Nurse Able standing next to you, chart in hand.

"This child doesn't look too good. I'm making him urgent."

Your eyebrows elevate a notch. A word of warning from a good ER nurse is worthy of careful consideration.

You glance at your wristwatch: fifteen minutes until the doctor replacing you comes on duty.

A child with fever is not what I need right now. Still, duty calls.

You manage a half smile at Nurse Able.

"Let me have the chart. I'll see the child now."

Vital signs on the chart show a temperature of 103°, pulse 120, respirations 20, blood pressure 112/72. The complaint listed is "fever and headache."

Up and off you go to the patient's room.

The youngster lies curled on his side on the stretcher. He's a thin, gangly lad, with short, curly, brown hair. He holds his hands on either side of his head, his eyes closed in a grimace.

The boy's mother sits in a chair next to the stretcher. Her posture is right-angled erect; her hands are folded on her lap. She wears a plain gray dress with a high, white collar.

"Tell me your concern about Abraham," you say.

She pauses before answering, reaching nervously to pat the bun of hair on the back of her head.

"His headache. It won't go away. His fever has been high. He started vomiting this morning. I think he's getting worse."

"How long has he been sick?"

"Five days. We've been praying he would get better. The whole congregation has prayed for him, but his fever won't break."

"Has Abraham had any tick bites in the past couple weeks?"

"No."

"Has he been exposed to anyone with a serious infection?"

"No. He's only been with his family and our church brethren."

You slide a stool to the head of the stretcher and sit down.

"Abraham, how are you feeling?" you ask softly.

The boy cracks open his eyes. "My head really hurts."

"Can you sit up for an exam?"

The lad props himself up on one elbow, then rises slowly to sitting.

"Can you put your chin here?" You place your index finger on the boy's upper chest, just below his neck.

Abraham moves his head down, but winces and stops before he bends his neck more than a few inches.

"I can't. It hurts," he says.

"Where?"

The boy puts his hand on the back of his neck.

You quickly examine the youngster. His throat is clear, his ears without infection, his heart and lung sounds normal, his abdomen soft.

Inspecting the boy's skin, you note several tiny maroon spots, the size of freckles, on his hands and forearms.

> **Question 1** — Possible causes of the boy's symptoms include:
> A) Viral (flu-like) illness.
> B) Viral meningitis.
> C) Bacterial meningitis.
> D) Rocky Mountain spotted fever.
> E) Tick-borne encephalitis.
> F) All of the above.
>
> **Answer** —
> F) is correct. Indeed, wise doctor — *all* of these infections are possibilities. Although many viral illnesses can cause mild fever and headache, the severity of the boy's headache, his stiff neck, and the skin rash all point toward the possibility of a serious illness such as meningitis.

Question 2 — You should recommend:
  A) Immediate lumbar puncture (spinal tap).
  B) Blood count and blood culture.
  C) Intravenous antibiotics.
  D) Calling a pediatrician.
  E) Admission to the hospital.
  F) All of the above.

Answer —
  F) is correct.

"Mrs. Alms, Abraham may have a serious infection such as meningitis. Meningitis is an infection around the brain and spinal cord. We need to start antibiotics and do a spinal tap at once. The risk of a spinal tap is very small. The benefits of knowing what kind of infection Abraham has may be lifesaving."

Mrs. Alms looks down at her hands in her lap. Her knuckles are white from pushing her palms together in prayer.

"Abraham's father and Pastor Ward are out in the waiting room. I need to talk to them before any treatment is given."

"If you want me to talk briefly with your husband, I'll be glad to. Meanwhile, the nurses and I are going to make preparations for the antibiotics and tests."

The mother rises from her seat. She puts a hand on Abraham's forehead.

"I'll be right back," she says. "I need to go talk to Papa."

The boy opens his eyes and closes them again, indicating his understanding. ❖

29

Religious Refusal

Your patient is: Abraham Alms, a 6 year-old with possible meningitis (infection around the brain).

The boy lies curled on his side on the stretcher. He holds his head in his hands, grimacing in pain.

"He's got fever, headache, and a skin rash," you tell the nurse in the room. "Stick an IV in, give him two grams of antibiotic, and we'll do a spinal tap. All lickety-split. His mother went to talk to the father and their pastor."

The door to the room opens. A solemn, bearded man, clothed in a white shirt and black suspenders, pants and shoes, steps into the room. The boy's mother, clad in similar plain, dark clothing, follows behind. Her eyes are cast down at her feet.

"No blood tests, no needles into the body," the man says. "I am the boy's father and I take responsibility for this decision. We have placed our faith in God. His will is our path. We will take the boy home and pray."

Question 1 — You should:
A) Consider a career in real estate.
B) Contact the hospital's lawyer.
C) Contact your own lawyer.
D) Make sure the father understands the implications of what he has said.
E) Let Mr. Alms take the boy home. The wishes of the family override your medical advice.

Answer —
D) is correct.

"Mr. Alms, Abraham might have meningitis, an infection around the brain. If he does, and you take him home, he will surely die. I give my strongest recommendation possible that you let us do tests and give antibiotics here in the hospital."

Abraham's father shakes his head back and forth.

"No. God's will shall be done. Our prayer is strong. If Abraham has a chance, it is through prayer. If he should die, he will be in heaven with God as a chosen one."

"Do you understand what I'm saying, what I recommend for Abraham?"

"I understand. It was a mistake that my wife brought my son to the hospital. But this is America, a country founded on religious freedom. Let us act on our beliefs and take Abraham home."

Question 2 — You should:

    A) Scream at the top of your lungs.

    B) Opt for early and immediate retirement.

    C) Ask the boy what he wants to do.

    D) Tell Mr. Alms his family's religious beliefs are overridden by your concerns for his son's health.

    E) Let Mr. Alms take the boy home. Personal and religious beliefs of the family override your medical advice.

Answer —

    D) is correct. If an *adult* patient is mentally competent (not insane, brain-injured, or under the influence of drugs or alcohol), he/she is allowed to make decisions about his/her own treatment. In the case of children, courts have generally ruled that a doctor should act in the interests of the child, regardless of the wishes of the parents.

"Mr. Alms, I'm sorry, but we have to go against your wishes. Abraham must stay here for treatment. He may die without it. I apologize that I cannot honor your beliefs."

Mr. Alms throws his shoulders back and puffs out his chest. His eyes fix you with an intense gaze.

"We take Abraham home," he says.

Mr. Alms turns, steps to the stretcher, lifts his son in his arms, and walks out the door of the treatment room.

Question 3 — You should immediately:
   A) Tackle Mr. Alms from behind.
   B) Tell the nurses to tackle Mr. Alms from behind while you grab the boy.
   C) Blast Mr. Alms with a sedative gun kept in the emergency department for unruly patients.
   D) Contact the hospital's lawyer to get a court order to treat the boy.
   E) Call hospital security personnel and local police to stop the father.

Answer —
   E) is correct. You must seek a court order to temporarily transfer guardianship of the child. However, in this situation, time is of the essence: You must begin treatment immediately in order to have a chance of saving the boy's life. ❖

Bleach Boy

Your patient is: 4 year-old Johnny Tuttle.

You hear the boy giggling as you enter the room. He's a whirling dervish, running to and fro. He stops to tug on his big sister, trying to pull her out of a chair. They're both light-skinned, topped with straight, flaxen hair.

The boy spies you. He pushes away from his sister and dashes to his mother, wrapping himself around her legs.

"Johnny, let loose and jump up on the stretcher so the doctor can examine you," his mother says.

The boy shakes his head back and forth. He buries his face in his mother's dark skirt.

"Mrs. Tuttle, how about if you sit on the stretcher and let Johnny sit in your lap," you suggest.

Johnny's mother lifts the boy underneath his arms. She sits on the stretcher and then eases Johnny onto her lap. The boy sits quietly, facing you, his motor on idle for now.

"He drank a swig or two of bleach," Mrs. Tuttle says.

"We're having our house painted," she explains. "The painters left some bleach in the garage in a Pepsi bottle. He got into it before I knew what was happening."

"How much do you think he drank?"

"Not more than a gulp or two."

"Are you sure?" you ask.

"Absolutely. I got the bottle away from him before he had a chance to drink more."

"Do you know if it was household bleach or industrial bleach?"

"The bleach came out of a white plastic jug, just like you buy at the store."

You Are the ER Doc!

"Household bleach, then. That's good," you say. "Has he vomited?"

"No."

"Has he complained of his throat or stomach burning?"

"No, he's acting like nothing happened. I'm the one who's a nervous wreck."

"Johnny, how do you feel?" you ask.

"Good," he replies.

"Does anything hurt?"

The boy shakes his head back and forth.

"Can you open your mouth and say, aaah?"

Johnny responds willingly, sticking his tongue out. His mouth and throat look moist and pink.

You press your stethoscope to Johnny's chest.

"Deep breaths, big guy." His lungs are clear.

Gently, you press inward with your fingers on the lad's abdomen.

"Nice and soft," you state.

Leaning close to the boy's face, you inhale steadily through your nose.

"I smell bleach, but just a whisper of a scent," you say.

Question 1 — You should:

A) Give the child some milk or juice to drink.

B) Radio for a helicopter to transport the boy to a Poison Treatment Center.

C) Get the boy ready for kidney dialysis since bleach will likely shut down his kidneys.

D) Warn the mother that Johnny might need an esophagus transplant if the bleach burned his esophagus.

E) Give Johnny syrup of ipecac to make him vomit.

F) Warn the mother that the bleach may turn the inside of Johnny's intestines white.

Answer —

A) is correct.

"Johnny, would you like some milk or juice?" you ask.

"Juice."

"Please," his mother urges.

"Pease," the boy says.

"Shouldn't we make him vomit or something?" Mrs. Tuttle says. "How about X-rays or blood tests?"

"Mrs. Tuttle, the only thing we need to do is dilute the bleach. To dilute the bleach, we'll give Johnny liquids to drink. It's as simple as that. He should be fine."

"Are you sure?" asks the mother.

"Cross my heart," you say, making an X over your left chest. "I know that common sense tells us that bleach might be harmful. But it turns out that regular household bleach is not dangerous, especially in small amounts. Of course, I wouldn't suggest drinking it on a regular basis."

Question 2 — You should recommend:

- A) Observation in the emergency department for three to four hours.
- B) Observation overnight in the hospital.
- C) Observation at home.
- D) Checking the house for other potentially hazardous ingestions.
- E) Checking the stools for white coloration the next several days.
- F) Both C) and D).

Answer —

F) is correct.

"Mrs. Tuttle, you can take Johnny home as soon as he drinks some juice. Watch him closely at home today. If you have any concerns, call me or bring him back to be checked again."

"I am so relieved, doctor. I thought drinking bleach would be a major problem."

"It could have been a big problem — if he had drunk something else. Other household products, like furniture cleaner or toilet bowl cleaner, can be very harmful if children swallow them.

Make sure anything harmful is out of Johnny's reach. This episode serves as a warning to make sure your house is child-proofed."

"I'll check my house as soon as I get home. And I'll let the painters know what happened, too."

"Please do. I'm sure the painters had no idea this could happen. Maybe we should all be a little more careful."

"Amen to that, doctor." ❖

Bugged

Your patient is: 57 year-old Wilbur Nunn.

"There's a durfball in Room 3 raising hell," reports Nurse Able. "Says he has a bug in his ear. He's one of the dirtiest patients I've seen in a long while. Can you go see him before he stinks up the whole place?"

"Another great case for me, eh?" you answer.

"There's a little boy next door in Room 4 with a cut on his eyebrow. His parents may leave if they have to put up with Mr. Skunk next door too long."

"See if you can put the little boy in another room. I'll go see Mr. Malodorous."

A minute later, you walk in Room 3.

"About time I got some service around here," says Mr. Nunn. "Got a bug in my ear and it's driving me crazy."

"How'd that happen?"

"I got kicked out of my rooming house. The places I'm sleeping now ain't too clean. I woke up with the bug in my ear this morning."

"Perhaps you were drinking a bit too much and passed out?"

"Durn it, doc, I don't need any lectures. I know what I am. Just get this bug out."

"All right, Mr. Nunn, let me have a look."

You put the otoscope in Mr. Nunn's ear and peer inside.

The stench of stale alcohol and body odor is thick. You hold your breath in an effort to keep the smell at bay.

Deep in the ear canal, up against Mr. Nunn's eardrum, sits a brownish insect.

"Little brown critter in there, Mr. Nunn. He's still alive, moving his legs."

YOU ARE THE ER DOC!

"I tell you, doc, it's driving me fruity. Get him out now, will you!"

Question 1 — You should:
- A) Tell Mr. Nunn he should go to the free clinic tomorrow since he has no money to pay his bill.
- B) Tell Mr. Nunn he smells too bad, and he must take a bath before you can treat him.
- C) Send Mr. Nunn to an ENT (Ear, Nose, and Throat) doctor tomorrow.
- D) Stick an instrument in Mr. Nunn's ear canal to get the bug out.
- E) Spray some lidocaine (numbing medicine) in Mr. Nunn's ear.

Answer —

E) is correct.

"Mr. Nunn, I'll be back in a minute. I need to get some medicine to spray in your ear."

"Damn it, doc, just reach in there with something and snatch the bug out."

"I don't want to do that, Mr. Nunn. If I put an instrument in your ear and you jump because it hurts, I might puncture your eardrum. Then we're in real trouble."

"What kind of medicine you gonna put in there?"

"Lidocaine. Numbing medicine, like we put in a syringe to numb the skin when we sew up cuts. Sometimes just spraying a little lidocaine in an ear canal will irritate the insect and make it crawl out."

"OK, just hurry up."

Minutes later, you are back in Room 3, Nurse Able in tow. Both of you wear paper surgical masks.

"Ready for surgery, doc?" Mr. Nunn asks.

"Not exactly," you answer. "Quite frankly, Mr. Nunn, the masks are to ward off the smell. Your hygiene is lacking at present."

Mr. Nunn looks puzzled. "Hygiene?" he says. "Oh, yeah. I haven't had a bath in a month."

"We noticed," Nurse Able responds.

Mr. Nunn laughs, displaying discolored nubs of teeth.

"You ready?" you ask Able.

"Ready."

"Lie back and look straight ahead at the ceiling, Mr. Nunn," you direct.

Mr. Nunn reclines. Rings of dirt and sweat from his neck smear the white pillowcase.

With a small syringe, you squirt the lidocaine into Mr. Nunn's ear canal.

Seconds later, a brown roach, the size of a pencil eraser, scurries out of Mr. Nunn's ear and plops onto the white pillow.

Thwack, goes a magazine onto the pillow.

Mr. Nunn jumps.

"Got him, Marshall Dillon," Able says.

"Nice shot, Able."

Another look into Mr. Nunn's ear: The ear canal is clear, the eardrum a normal, pearly white.

"That takes care of your problem, Mr. Nunn."

"Yeah, thanks, doc. But while you're here, can you look at one more thing real quick? I think that I've got worms in my intestine."

Question 2 — You should:

A) Tell Mr. Nunn he should go to the free clinic tomorrow since he has no money to pay his bill.

B) Tell Mr. Nunn he smells too bad, and must take a bath before you can treat him further.

C) Send Mr. Nunn to a specialist, a gastroenterologist (stomach/intestine) doctor.

D) Assign the rest of Mr. Nunn's care to Nurse Able.

E) Check Mr. Nunn further, assuming you have no pressing emergencies with other patients.

Answer —

E) is correct. You didn't go into emergency medicine for the money.

"OK, Mr. Nunn. What's the next problem?"

Mr. Nunn pulls his dirt-and-food-stained t-shirt up, exposing his ample abdomen.

"Something's in there, doc, crawling around. I can feel them sometimes. I think they're crawling out of my insides. They come out my bellybutton."

With gloved hands, you spread back the folds of fat around Mr. Nunn's bellybutton. In the dark hole, white worms squirm slowly back and forth.

The sight before your eyes takes several seconds to register in your brain.

"Maggots, Mr. Nunn. You have maggots in your umbilicus."

Fighting off a wave of nausea, you glance at Nurse Able, standing at the head of the stretcher, out of Mr. Nunn's line-of-sight.

Weird, she mouths the single word, shaking her head back and forth.

Question 3 — You should:

A) Call Ace Pest Control and Exterminating Company.

B) Say, "Yes, too darn weird for me!" and run out of the room.

C) Say, "I am utterly and totally grossed out," and "It's your case from here on, Nurse Able."

D Clean the maggots out of Mr. Nunn's bellybutton.

E) Refer Mr. Nunn to a specialist in parasites to remove the maggots and check for inside-the-body maggots.

Answer —

D) is correct. You don't practice emergency medicine if you have a weak stomach.

"Able, hand me some alcohol and gauze, would you?"

"My pleasure," she replies, stifling a gag.

You pour alcohol into Mr. Nunn's umbilicus. Nurse Able holds back the folds of fat on Mr. Nunn's belly while you swipe the area with gauze. Ten or twelve maggots come out before you see that the bottom of the cavern is empty and sealed.

"The maggots were in your bellybutton, Mr. Nunn, not inside your abdomen."

Question 4 — You should:

A) Ask Mr. Nunn, "Any more bugs in your system?"

B) Ask Mr. Nunn, "Any more interesting problems for me to treat?"

C) Put Mr. Nunn in the hospital since he is clearly not taking care of himself.

D) Refer Mr. Nunn to a free medical clinic for ongoing medical care.

E) Recommend Mr. Nunn contact AA (Alcoholics Anonymous).

F) Get a social worker to try to help Mr. Nunn with his housing and hygiene needs.

G) A), B), and C) are correct.

H) D), E), and F) are correct.

Answer —

H) is correct. Mr. Nunn needs help. Realistically, though, Mr. Nunn has to want to change before anyone will make headway in helping him. ❖

Taillight Sign

Your patient is: Emma Olner, an 88 year-old female.

The complaint on the chart reads: *sick, hurting.*

Mrs. Olner lies on the stretcher, her back raised at a 45-degree angle. She rests quietly, her eyes closed. Snow-white hair in a disheveled bun tops her head.

A worn, blue suitcase sits on the floor, beside the stretcher.

"Mrs. Olner," you begin.

The old lady opens her eyes and inspects you through trifocals. The lenses of the glasses are smudged with fingerprints.

"Hello, doctor."

"What brings you to the Emergency Department?"

"My son, Ronnie."

"No, I meant what kind of problem?"

"I guess they thought I needed to come."

"Who's they?"

"Ronnie. And his wife, Rita. I stay with them. They take care of me."

"What do *you* think? Is anything bothering you?"

"No."

"Are you hurting anywhere?"

"In my back."

"When did that begin?"

"Oh, 10 or 15 years ago. I've got osteoporosis, you know."

"Are you having any new symptoms?"

"My bowels aren't moving like they should."

"When did that begin?"

"I've had that all my life."

Question 1 — You should :

A) Examine Mrs. Olner.

B) Talk to the family.

C) Ask medical records to send down the charts of Mrs. Olner's past admissions.

D) Consult your crystal ball and ouija board for help.

E) Call in a gerontologist (a specialist in treating elderly patients) to figure out what is wrong with Mrs. Olner.

F) A), B), and C).

Answer —

F) is correct. All three actions might help.

"Able, can you locate Mrs. Olner's family?" you ask your nurse. "I need to ask them why they brought her in."

"Not possible," Able answers.

"Why not?"

"They've fled the scene. Outa' here. Adios, amigos. A classic case, I'd call it."

"A classic case? What do you mean?"

"A Granny Drop. Also known as a positive Taillight Sign. When the family wants a weekend off from caring for an elderly person, they drop the aged one off at the ER, then speed off into the sunset before anyone can ask them questions. The only view you get of the family is the taillights of their car fading into the distance."

"Mrs. Olner's family really left?"

"Yep. And in case you missed it, Mrs. Olner also has a positive Suitcase Sign — the family packed her suitcase so she can stay at the Hometown Hospital Hilton a few days."

You shake your head in disbelief, yet recognize that Nurse Able speaks from her thousands-of-shifts experience in the emergency department.

You proceed to examine Mrs. Olner. Physically, she is fine. Mentally, her mind wanders. You cannot deem her responsible for her own self-care.

You Are the ER Doc!

Question 2 — You should:

A) Call Mrs. Olner's doctor and suggest that Mrs. Olner be admitted to the hospital for social reasons.

B) Call Mrs. Olner's doctor and make up an emergency medical condition requiring admission to the hospital, a reason that Medicare will accept to pay for the admission.

C) Call the police to come pick up Mrs. Olner.

D) Send the patient to a local shelter for the homeless.

E) Notify the Highway Patrol to arrest the family and bring them back to the emergency department.

Answer —

A) is correct.

"I've got Dr. Jones on the phone," says the unit secretary.

"Dr. Jones, I've got one of your patients here, 88 year-old Emma Olner. Nothing new with her, but her family dropped her here and took off. She's unable to take care of herself. If we send her home, I'm afraid she might burn down the house or something. There's no way we can get social services to find her a sitter at 9 P.M. on a Friday night. And, if we send her to a homeless persons' shelter, someone might take advantage of her."

A deep sigh emanates from the other end of the phone.

"Her family has done this twice before," reports Dr. Jones. "By the time social services finds a sitter or a nursing home bed, Mrs. Olner's family shows up and reclaims the old lady."

"Then you'll admit her?"

"Yes, I will. Medicare may not pay, but we still have to think of the patient first. At least for now, we need to protect her by putting her in the hospital. I will ask social services to investigate the home situation, though. This is a form of negligence."

"I agree. Thank you for putting the patient first, Dr. Jones."

Nice job, doctor. Sometimes the emergency department is the dumping ground for society's problems. Yet, you must uphold the physician's golden rule: Always act in the best interests of the patient! ❖

Squirrel Bite

Your patient is: Timmy Long, a 7 year-old bitten by a squirrel.

The boy sits on the stretcher reading a comic book, blowing a pink bubble with his gum. Strands of brown hair flop over his ears and onto his forehead.

Timmy's mother sits stiffly in a chair beside the stretcher, holding her purse on her lap.

"How did you get bitten?" you ask.

"We've been feeding squirrels in our back yard. One of them thought my finger was a peanut, I guess."

"Where did the squirrel bite you?"

Timmy holds out his arm, palm up, and extends his index finger. His face glows with pride as he displays pinpoint-sized, red marks on his fingertip.

You hold Timmy's finger in between your index finger and thumb, inspecting the digit.

"Did it break the skin? Did it bleed?"

"A little bit."

The mother shifts in her seat. "I'm worried about rabies, doctor. I've heard people can die from rabies."

Question 1 — You should:
- A) Quarantine the boy for six weeks to see if he acts rabid.
- B) Call for assistance to help hold the boy down so you can administer a dozen rabies shots into the stomach.
- C) Cut out the area of the wound so infection won't set in.
- D) Reassure the mother and patient that there is no risk of rabies.

Answer —

D) is correct. Squirrels are rodents, and rodents do not pass rabies (at least in the United States*). A bite from a bat, fox, or raccoon would be a different story, a definite cause for concern about rabies.

"I think you'll make it another hundred years or so, big guy," you tell the boy, rubbing the shock of hair on his head.

"Does he need a tetanus shot, doctor?" the mother says. "He had one just before starting school last year."

Question 2 — You should:

A) Whip a tetanus shot out of your pocket and stick it in the boy's arm before he realizes what is happening.

B) Ask if the boy has been good or bad before deciding on giving a shot.

C) Tell the mother that tetanus shots cover small wounds like this for at least ten years.

D) Advise that tetanus and lockjaw are only a problem with wounds from rusty nails.

Answer —

C) is correct. Tetanus boosters prevent lockjaw for at least ten years on minor wounds and for at least five years on major, dirty wounds. *Any* wound that breaks the skin (not just cuts from rusty nails) can pass tetanus germs and cause lockjaw, an often fatal illness.

"You mean I don't need a shot, doctor?" Timmy asks.
"No, Timmy, you don't. Did you clean the cut yet?"
"My mom made me wash my hands and so did the nurse."
"Great. Washing with regular soap and water is one of the best ways to get germs out of a wound. But, Mrs. Long, you'll still need to watch Timmy closely."

Medical note: In medicine, as in life, exceptions to rules are common. Beavers, which are actually large rodents, have been found to be rabid in the United States.

Question 3 — Timmy's mother should watch for:
A) A sudden craving for nuts.
B) Acorn breath.
C) Increased tree-climbing activity.
D) "Squirrely" behavior of any type.
E) Infection in the wound.

Answer —

E) is correct. *Any* animal bite wound (squirrel, monkey, dog, man, giraffe, etc.) is a contaminated wound, at higher risk for infection. Animals have millions of bacteria (germs) in their mouth. When an animal bite breaks the skin, germs are pushed into the normally germ-free layers beneath the skin. There, the bacteria can multiply rapidly, causing infection. Deep and large bite wounds have an increased chance of infection compared to small,shallow wounds.

"So long, big guy. Slap me five, will you?" you tell Timmy.
"Mrs. Long, bring Timmy back if he develops signs of infection: pus, increasing redness, warmth, and swelling of the bite area, or red streaks spreading from the wound."

Timmy Long is discharged from the emergency department. Another save. Nice going, doctor! ❖

Fox Lick

Your patient is: Phyllis Jango, a 10 year-old who has been licked by a fox.

The girl sits on the stretcher, her gaze fixed on a Nancy Drew mystery in her hands. Her father sits in a chair next to the girl, peering through reading glasses at a copy of *The Wall Street Journal*.

"Good book?" you ask.

The girl looks up and nods her head.

"What's this I hear about you being licked by a fox?"

"I was at Camp Treetops yesterday. We hiked into Sandhills State Park. A little fox was running around in the woods, kind of going in circles. We caught it and when I picked it up, it licked my hands, that's all."

"The fox let you pick it up?"

"Yeah, it didn't seem afraid at all. But it had a glazed look in its eyes, so I put it back down and it ran off."

"Hmm," you reply. "Can I see your hands?"

The girl extends her arms.

Small red lines criss-cross the backs of her hands.

"Those scratches on your hands, how did you get them?"

"Picking berries yesterday morning."

"Before the fox licked you?"

"Uh-huh."

"Doctor, do we really need to worry?" the girl's father interjects. "The camp nurse said we should bring Phyllis here as a precaution since rabies has been reported in wild animals in our county. But it's not like the fox bit her or even scratched her."

amazon.com.

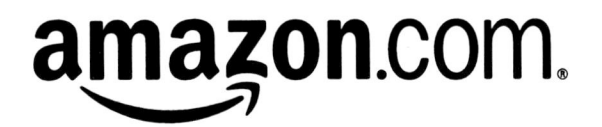

http://www.amazon.com

Billin
Denr
3428 Hunte
Stow,
Unit

Shippir
Denr
3428 Hunte
Stow,
Unit

Your order of December 2, 2001 (Order ID 102-5033811-8952951)

Qty	Item
	In This Shipment
1	You are the ER Doc! True-to Life Cases for You to Treat (P-1-B11B56)

This shipment co

You can track the status of this order, and all your recent orders, online b
Returns are easy -- even for gifts! Visit http://www

Thanks for shopping at Ama

131/buuu14144/-1-/1vdf/SMART_MAIL/1195/std-us/1410619/1202-22:40/1202-23:03

Address:
is Haver
's Crossing Dr.
OH 44224
d States

g Address:
is Haver
's Crossing Dr.
OH 44224
d States

amazon.com.

Amazon.com
1850 Mercer Rd.
Lexington, KY 40511

Dennis Haver
3428 Hunter's Crossing Dr.
Stow, OH 44224
United States

buuu14144/-1-/1195/std-us/1410619/330-677-9385

SMART_MAI

1

Description	Format	Our Price	Total
Unknown	Paperback	$11.95	$11.95

Subtotal		$11.95
Shipping & Handling		$3.99
Order Total		$15.94
Paid via Visa		$15.94
Balance Due		$0.00

npletes your order.

visiting "Your Account" page at http://www.amazon.com/your-account.

amazon.com/returns and save a trip to the post office.

on.com, and please come again!

Earth's Biggest Selection

Question 1 — Chances of rabies being transmitted to Phyllis are:

A) Almost 100%.

B) 50%.

C) About the same as the chance of Phyllis transmitting rabies to the fox.

D) Very small.

E) Zero.

Answer —

D) is correct.

"We have to be concerned about the possibility of rabies, however small," you tell the father. "A bite from a bat, skunk, raccoon, fox, or domestic cat is the most common way rabies is transmitted to humans. Even without a bite, though, if saliva from a rabid animal enters a person's bloodstream, rabies can be spread. The scratches on Phyllis's hands mean that the fox could have passed the rabies virus to her just by licking her hands."

"The fox wasn't foaming at the mouth or trying to bite people, though," the father responds.

"No, but the fox's behavior was abnormal. Foxes don't normally let humans pick them up. Strange behavior of any type raises the concern that an animal is rabid."

"Rabies is bad news, isn't it, doctor?"

Question 2 — The rabies virus is:

A) Not a big deal.

B) Like the swine flu virus (mild).

C) More deadly than the virus causing AIDS.

D) Fatal unless treatment is started as soon as symptoms occur.

Answer —

C) is correct.

"Mr. Jango, rabies is a fatal disease. The only effective treatment is giving preventive vaccine and antibody shots. If we wait until a person shows symptoms of rabies, then it's too late."

Mr. Jango squints his eyes shut, shakes his head, then opens his eyes again.

"Rabies shots. Isn't that thirteen painful shots into the stomach or something?"

"Not any more. We give two shots the first day, then four more shots over the next 28 days. The shots are given into the arm, and they don't hurt any more than other immunization shots."

"We have no choice, do we?"

"No. You don't want to take the chance, albeit tiny, of Phyllis getting rabies. Her life would be at risk."

"OK. Let's get started with the shots," the father says.

"Do you understand, Phyllis?"

"I have to get shots so I don't get rabies or else I might die."

"That's it in a nutshell. We'll make it as easy as we can." ❖

Granny's Pain

Your patient is: Zelda Phipps, an 83 year-old lady with pain in the right side of her chest.

"It hurts bad, doctor. I haven't had pain like this since I had a kidney stone some 30 years ago. Or since I had my babies longer ago than I can remember."

Mrs. Phipps grimaces, the wrinkles on her forehead deepening below her silver hair. She reaches with her left hand under her right armpit all the way onto her right upper back. "Hurts all the way 'round, from front to back."

"Just on the right side?" you ask.

"Only on the right."

"Any fever or cough or shortness of breath?"

"No, just the pain. Just this awful, burning pain."

"Let's take a listen to your lungs, Mrs. Phipps."

First on the left side of her chest, then on the right, you listen. Her lungs move air in and out like a bellows, normally.

"Your lungs sound fine." Taking the stethoscope from your ears, you add, "When did these bumps come up on your skin?"

"The day after the pain came on. Started with just one little patch, then more patches came the next day or two."

"They look like tiny blisters, don't they?"

"That's right where the pain is the worst, too."

Question 1 — Mrs. Phipps has:
    A) An infection.
    B) A herpes infection.
    C) An infection with the chickenpox virus.
    D) A problem with her nerves.
    E) Shingles.
    F) All of the above.

Answer —
   F) is correct.

"Mrs. Phipps, you have shingles. It's an infection with the herpes zoster virus that gave you chickenpox as a child. The virus laid quiet in the nerves of your body all these years. Sometimes it comes out along a few nerve bands on one side of the body, usually on the chest, causing shingles."
"I've heard of shingles, but I didn't know it was the chickenpox virus. My sister, Mildred, had shingles a couple years ago, and she liked to have never got rid of it. Still gives her a fit from time to time, I believe."

Question 2 — You can tell Mrs. Phipps she can:
   A) Expect a miracle cure with one shot.
   B) Take some medicine by mouth which will make the shingles go away quickly.
   C) Have pain for a couple more days at most.
   D) Take some medicine which might help the shingles go away quicker, but she may have pain for weeks or months.

Answer —
   D) is correct.

"Mrs. Phipps, our antibiotics against viruses aren't very effective. I'm going to prescribe medicine which can help the rash go away quicker, but you may still hurt for weeks or perhaps even months."
"Can you give me some pain pills, too, doctor?"
"You bet. I'll prescribe some pain pills, but be careful — they make you groggy, and they'll tend to constipate you, too."
"Hurtin' like fire and stopped up, too, is that what you're telling me?"
"I'm afraid so, Mrs. Phipps, but I want to be honest on what you're facing. Shingles doesn't kill people, but it surely is painful. You're going to need some support from your family and friends to get through this."

"I'll make it doctor, if they're all as good to me as you've been."

Good care, doctor. Remember — if you can't cure, at least comfort. And, sometimes a simple thank-you or compliment is enough to make your job worthwhile. ❖

You Are the ER Doc!

Handy Dandy

Your patient is: Stuart Jamison III, a 24 year-old male with an injured hand.

Mr. Jamison sits on the stretcher, looking as if he had just stepped off a yacht. He's clad in a green polo shirt, tan pants, and brown boating shoes. His dark hair is stylishly groomed. A gold necklace highlights the tanned skin inside his shirt collar.

A young lady with straight, down-to-the waist, blond hair stands next to him. She rubs his back with her left hand.

"Doctor, how are you?" the young man says.

"Fine, Mr. Jamison. And you?"

"Good, except for my hand. It hurts like the dickens."

Mr. Jamison flashes a grin. You note a quarter-sized bruise under his left cheekbone.

He extends his right hand, gingerly supported by his left hand underneath. A one-inch cut, a red crescent, shines on the knuckle of his little finger. The top of his hand and little finger, above and below the cut, are red and swollen.

"I hit my hand on a door two days ago," he says. "Since then, it's become rather painful and swollen."

"It looks like it hurts," you acknowledge. "Flip your hand over so I can see your palm. Put both hands palm up, side-by-side."

The young man rotates his hands slowly. The palm of his right hand is puffy. The palm creases, easily visible on his left hand, are absent on the right. The little finger on the right hand is puffed like a sausage.

"Can you straighten your little finger?"

"I'll try."

Mr. Jamison narrows his eyes and scrunches his face. He straightens the index, middle, and ring fingers of his right hand. His little finger doesn't budge an inch.

"I can't," he relates. "It hurts too much."

Question 1 — You should ask:
   A) If pus has come from the wound; if Mr. Jamison has had fever or chills.
   B) The date of Mr. Jamison's last tetanus booster shot.
   C) If Mr. Jamison has any serious underlying illnesses.
   D) How Mr. Jamison really hurt his hand.
   E) All of the above.

Answer —
   E) is correct.

"Has any pus drained from the wound?" you ask.

"Thick, yellow stuff filled the cut today. I cleaned it out with peroxide before I came in."

"Have you had any fever or chills?"

Mr. Jamison's blond companion speaks up. "His temperature was normal. I took it three times."

"When was your last tetanus booster?"

"When I was 14. I cut my foot when I was fishing for marlin on my old man's boat."

"Do you have any serious medical problems which could affect your ability to fight infection? Diabetes? AIDS? Cancer?"

Mr. Jamison turns to face his blond cohort. "Do I have any of those?" he says.

"You better not."

"I'm healthy as a horse, doctor," Mr. Jamison says.

"Do you overuse alcohol? Any drug use?" you ask.

"I drink some, but not excessively. I've never used drugs."

"The next question is important. Take your time to answer." You pause to let your words to sink in.

"Did you really hurt your hand punching a door? Or, did you punch a person and cut your hand on someone's tooth? If that's the case, your cut is the same as a bite wound. Bite wounds are heavily contaminated with mouth germs. The wounds get infected easily and are treated with different antibiotics than regular wounds."

The young man looks at his friend.

"Better tell him the truth," she says.

Mr. Jamison turns back toward you. "You're right, I hit someone," he says. "We were having a few beers at Red Dog's Pub. Somebody made a less-than-nice comment to my lady here. I told the man to mind his own business. The next thing I know he and I were going a few rounds in the parking lot. He looks worse than I do, I'll tell you that."

"So you cut your hand on somebody's mouth."

"Yes sir. Just the same, I'd rather my parents not know about that part."

"What you've told me is part of your medical record. No one has access to your chart unless you give permission. What you tell your parents or anyone else is your business. You're 24 years-old."

"OK. Now that you know how I cut my hand, can you just give me an antibiotic or something and I'll be on my way?"

Question 2 — You should recommend:

A) A tetanus booster shot.

B) Keeping the hand elevated to decrease swelling.

C) Intravenous antibiotics.

D) Calling a doctor who treats hand injuries to evaluate Mr. Jamison for surgery.

E) All of the above.

Answer —

E) is correct.

"Mr. Jamison, you have a serious infection. It can't be treated with just an antibiotic by mouth. Your infection extends deep into the middle of the palm and fingers. That area of the hand contains tendons which control the fingers. We need to call a hand surgeon to drain the pus from your hand. You also need intravenous antibiotics and a tetanus booster shot."

"Sounds like fun," Mr. Jamison says sarcastically. "Any other tortures you can think of?"

"Keep the hand elevated above your heart to help minimize the swelling."

"I'll make sure Stuart elevates his hand, doctor," his companion says. She places Mr. Jamison's hand gently atop her shoulder. "You can just be my handy dandy for now," she says.

"Cool, babe," Mr. Jamison says. "I'll keep my hand up as long as I get to hang it on you." ❖

You Are the ER Doc!

Fever in a Four Year-Old

Your patient is: Tommy Tuttle, a 4 year-old with high fever.

Tommy sits on the stretcher, his attention riveted to a coloring book. The boy's hand jumps back and forth with a crayon, like a seismograph needle during an earthquake.

"Tonya! Trevor! Quit that." Tommy's mother tells the other children in the room, each trying to wrestle a toy pickup truck away from the other.

You smile. "Got your hands full, it looks like."

"More than full," she says.

"Tell me what concerns you about Tommy. The chart says he's had a fever of 104 degrees at home. It's 102.8 right now."

"He's had fever since yesterday morning. I can't seem to break it. His temperature goes down to 100 with Tylenol, but it's right back up four hours later."

"Any other symptoms? Cough? Vomiting or diarrhea? Ear pain or sore throat? Headache?"

"No, nothing else."

"How's he eating?"

"His appetite's a little bit off, but he's drinking lots of fluids."

"That's good. Fluids help control fever, too."

Turning your attention to the boy, you continue.

"How are you feeling right now, Tommy?"

"Fine."

"Do you hurt anyplace?"

The boy cocks his head to one side, thinking.

"No."

"Throat and ears feel OK?"

"Uh-huh."

"Are you hungry right now?"

"Mom promised me McDonald's if I'm good. I want a cheeseburger and fries."

"How about sitting here with your legs over the side of the bed so I can take a look at you?"

The boy closes his coloring book and slides forward.

You hold a penlight in your hand and move it back and forth.

"Follow the light," you say.

The boy moves his head to and fro. His chin comes down on his chest without difficulty as you touch the light to his abdomen.

No neck stiffness. No sign of meningitis.

The boy's ears and throat look normal. His lungs are clear, his heart sounds are good, his belly is soft. He has no skin rash.

Normal exam.

Question 1 — You should:

A) Get a urine specimen by catheterization to check for urinary tract infection.

B) Order a blood count and blood culture.

C) Do a lumbar puncture (spinal tap).

D) Start intravenous antibiotics as soon as the specimens for the tests are obtained.

E) Call a pediatrician to see the child; admit the child to the hospital.

F) None of the above.

Answer —

F) is correct.

"Mrs. Tuttle," you begin, "I don't see any sign of a serious infection. No hint of meningitis, Rocky Mountain spotted fever, pneumonia, or even a throat or ear infection. Tommy very likely has a viral infection."

"The only test," you continue, "we need to do is a urinalysis. Tommy can urinate in a specimen container. We'll check it in a jiffy, just to make sure he's not hiding a kidney infection."

"His fever is so high, though. Don't you need to do an X-ray? Can you give him an antibiotic?"

"What's important is not how high the fever is, but what other symptoms he has along with the fever. Tommy has no other symptoms of concern. All the X-rays in the world wouldn't tell us anything. And, an antibiotic won't help, since they work against bacterial infections, not viruses."

"What should I do?"

"Exactly what you're doing now. Be a good mother. Watch Tommy closely. Give him Tylenol or ibuprofen for fever. If he gets worse, bring him back or see your pediatrician at once."

Mrs. Tuttle stands up and puts both hands on the stretcher. She looks at Tommy and sighs.

"Times like these make me wonder about the wisdom of having children."

"I can identify with that," you reply. "But the good times outweigh the bad, don't they?"

She turns and manages a smile.

"Yes, they do, doctor. Yes, they do." ❖

A Baby with Fever

Your patient is: Simon Smidge, a 2 month-old with fever.

Nurse Jones hands you a chart. "A wee-little one with a temperature," she says.

"I'm on the way," you answer, striding toward Room 9.

Simon lies sleeping in his mother's arms.

His mother sits in a chair, rocking her son. Brown hair in the shape of an inverted U frames her face. Dark eyes solicit you with a mother's concern.

You sit on a stool opposite mother and child.

"Tell me your main concern about Simon."

"He's had fever, and he won't eat."

"When did the fever start, and how high has it been?"

"This morning. It was 102 degrees an hour ago."

"Any other symptoms? Vomiting, diarrhea, cough, skin rash?"

"Nothing like that. He's been sleeping more, though."

"Let's do a quick exam. Keep Simon in your arms. We'll try not to disturb him more than we have to."

The vital signs on the chart read: Temperature 101.9 (rectal), pulse 134, respirations 30, blood pressure 98/66.

Vital signs good, except for the temperature.

The child breathes easily. His overall appearance is normal, except for his skin, which is mottled pink and white instead of uniform pink.

Running your hand gently over the fine hair on Simon's scalp, you feel for the soft spot on top of his head. Your fingers locate it and probe gently; it's soft and slightly indented.

Normal. No sign of increased pressure inside the head.

You place a stethoscope on the infant's chest: Normal heart

beat. No heart murmur. Lungs clear.

The abdomen is soft when your hand presses on it. You pull loose the tape on the child's diaper, then pull back the front of the white plastic.

Genitals normal, both testicles down, no bulge of a hernia.

Checking the skin on the chest, stomach, back, palms and soles, no rash is visible.

The child hasn't stirred a bit. Too sleepy!

"Let's check his ears and throat," you say. "We'll see if he tolerates it in your arms. If he squirms too much, we'll have to hold him down."

The child's eardrums are a normal pearly-white color. His throat is clear. What *is* unusual is that Simon doesn't wake up with the ear or throat exam, even when a tongue blade is pressed on his tongue to open his mouth.

Question 1 — You should:

   A) Get a urine specimen by catheterization to check for urinary tract infection.
   B) Order a blood count and blood culture.
   C) Do a lumbar puncture (spinal tap).
   D) Start intravenous antibiotics promptly.
   E) Call a pediatrician to see the child and admit the child to the hospital.
   F) All of the above.

Answer—

F) is correct.

"Mrs. Smidge," you begin, "we have to be very careful with a child Simon's age when fever is present. Just like older children, an infant can get fever from a viral infection or a bacterial infection. The problem is, in an infant, differentiating between a relatively harmless viral infection and a serious bacterial infection is difficult. We need to assume and treat for a whole-body bacterial infection until we know otherwise."

"Will he be OK?"

"I don't think he's in any big danger right now. If we act quickly and decisively, there's a very good chance he'll be fine."

"What can I do to help, doctor?"

"What you're doing now. Continue being a good mother and giving him every comfort you can."

Two weeks later, you get a report from Simon's hospitalization. Tests showed pyelonephritis, an infection in the kidneys. Simon was successfully treated with intravenous antibiotics.

Way to go, doctor. Always remember: Fever in an infant is a matter to be taken seriously. ❖

You Are the ER Doc!

Moped Malady

Your patient is: Deever Grant, a 55 year-old male with a cut on his face.

The chart states, *Driving a Moped, ran off the road and hit a parked school bus.*
"Hey, doc!" Mr. Grant greets you.
The smell of alcohol and body odor wafts from him in noxious waves.
"Mr. Grant, how are you?" you answer. You take a step back and try not to breathe too deeply.
"Couldn't be better, doc. 'Cept for this little cut on my face." Mr. Grant raises his hand to his forehead. His fingers trace a large gash, three inches long, curving over his left eyebrow.

Question 1 — You should:
- A) Check Mr. Grant for neck injuries first.
- B) Check Mr. Grant's brain function.
- C) Check Mr. Grant for serious internal injuries which may not be obvious.
- D) Check Mr. Grant's cut only after checking the above.
- E) Make sure Mr. Grant has had a tetanus booster shot in the past ten years.
- F) All of the above.

Answer —
- F) is correct. Suspect the worst (spine or brain injury) but hope for the best (just a cut). Hidden, unsuspected injury is sometimes difficult to detect in an intoxicated patient.

"Does this hurt?" You tap on the back of Mr. Grant's neck with your fist.

"Nope."

"Put your chin down on your chest, Mr. Grant."

Mr. Grant flexes his neck, touching his chin to his chest.

"Let me check your pupil reaction." The black orbs in the center of Mr. Grant's eyes shrink briskly to bright light shined in them.

A dozen tests and several minutes later, you tell Mr. Grant, "Everything looks fine inside of you. No sign of an internal injury. Your brain is working fine."

"Musta' done me some good running into that bus, doc. My brain ain't worked too good for a long time." Mr. Grant grins and cackles, laughing himself into a fit of coughing.

Question 2 — You should:

A) Put a "butterfly" bandage on Mr. Grant's cut and send him home.

B) Use metal staples to close Mr. Grant's wound.

C) Use catgut sutures (stitches) to close Mr. Grant's wound.

D) Send Mr. Grant to see a plastic surgeon the next day.

E) Discuss with Mr. Grant whether you or a plastic surgeon should sew up his cut promptly.

Answer —

E) is correct. A butterfly bandage will not work on a large wound. Staples leave a bigger scar, so they should not be used on the face. The wound needs to be closed now, with nylon sutures. Either you or a plastic surgeon should repair the wound.

"Mr. Grant, you have a big gash on your forehead that needs to be sewn up. I'm an emergency doctor. We see everything, from colds to cuts to heart attacks. I can sew up your cut, or we can call a plastic surgeon. A plastic surgeon has had special training in wound repair, so your scar might be less visible. Also, I've got a lot of other patients to take care of, so it might be several hours

You Are the ER Doc!

before I could get your wound closed."

"Call the plastic surgeon, doc. I want to stay beautiful, know what I mean?" Mr. Grant smiles widely, exhibiting the few remaining teeth in his mouth.

A few minutes later, the ward secretary says, "Pick up line two, doctor, it's Dr. Paisley calling you back."

"Dr. Paisley," you begin, "I've got a 55 year-old male who ran into a bus while driving a Moped. He's got a three-inch laceration on his forehead. Can you come and sew him up?"

"Is he drunk?"

"He's been drinking, yes."

"Does he have insurance?"

"I'm not sure, let me check his chart," you answer. A glance at Mr. Grant's chart reveals the answer. "No, no insurance."

"Can't help you," comes the response. A click and then dial tone greets your ears through the phone.

Question 3 — You should:
  A) Tell Mr. Grant the plastic surgeon is operating at another hospital and too busy to come sew him up.
  B) Call Ann Landers for advice.
  C) Call the plastic surgeon back and threaten him with a large fine and jail sentence if he doesn't come in.
  D) Give the patient a knock-out drug, suture the wound yourself, but tell him the plastic surgeon fixed the cut.
  E) Tell the patient what happened and let him decide what to do.

Answer —
  E) is correct. C) is an option, too, if you think a plastic surgeon is essential. According to federal law, an on-call doctor must respond to treat a patient in need, or risk fine and/or imprisonment.

"Mr. Grant, the plastic surgeon doesn't want to come in," you say. "We can try to find another plastic surgeon if you like, but chances are slim. The other option is for me to fix your cut as time allows."

"You fix it, doc. You do a lot of sewing on people, right?"

"That I do, Mr. Grant."

"You'll be fine then."

"I appreciate your vote of confidence, Mr. Grant. You can be sure I'll take my time and do a good job. Right now, though, I've got to go see a patient with chest pain. I'll get back in as soon as I can."

You spin around and stride toward the patient with chest pain. Nurse Able steps in beside you.

"Too bad you can't refuse treatment, too," she whispers.

"I don't know any emergency doctor that would," you answer. "Nor would any emergency nurse, for that matter."

"Right," Able answers, "we see them all." ❖

You Are the ER Doc!

Reptile GI Blues

Your patient is: Ginger Meeks, a 4 year-old with diarrhea.

"Doctor, you've got to do something. She's had diarrhea for five straight days."

Ginger's mother greets you with these words. She stands next to the stretcher, wringing a wet washcloth in her hands. She pauses to lay it on her daughter's head.

"I'm worried she's dehydrated."

Ginger lies quietly on the stretcher. Curlets of blonde hair circle her pale face. The color is gone from her lips. The girl's blue eyes track your every move.

"Let's see what's going on," you tell the mother.

Turning your attention to the little girl, you pull up a stool and sit down, your face at her level.

"How do you feel, Ginger?"

"OK."

"Do you hurt anywhere?"

The little girl shakes her head no.

"Have you been throwing up?"

A nod of the head up and down.

Question 1 — You should:

A) Ask the little girl more questions.

B) Ask the mother more questions.

C) Ask the nurse to start IV fluids immediately.

D) Order a stool culture, blood tests and urinalysis.

E) Call a pediatrician to see the child.

Answer —

    B) is probably the best choice. Establishing initial rapport with a patient is important, even when the patient is a child. You've done so, talking face-to-face with Ginger. And, while you do need to examine the little girl, a few other questions need to be asked first.

Turning to the mother, you query further.
"Has she vomited?"
"Twice today. She can't keep any fluids down."
"Any fever?"
"A little. No higher than 101 degrees."
"Any blood in the stool?"
"Yesterday, she had an accident in her pants. She hasn't done that since potty-training at age two. There were streaks of red on her underpants."
"Anyone else sick at home? Are any of the children she plays with sick?"
"Nobody else is sick."
"Did she eat anything unusual?"
"No. She ate the same things we did."
You proceed with your exam.
The vital signs on the chart show a temperature of 101.5, a pulse of 130, normal blood pressure and respirations.
Overall, Ginger looks "green around the gills." Her eyes lack sparkle; dark rings surround her orbs. The mucous membranes inside her mouth are sticky and dry, not glistening with moisture as normal. Her abdomen is soft to touch. When you press on her tummy with your hand, Ginger does not grimace or cry out in pain.

    Question 2 — The most likely causes of the girl's symptoms include:

    A) Viral infection.

    B) Bacterial infection.

    C) Food poisoning.

    D) Faking illness to get out of school.

    E) Maternal hysteria.

Answer —

A) and B) are most likely. Food poisoning is unlikely, since others ate the same food as the little girl, and they are not ill. Bacterial infection is more likely than viral infection in this case: Fever, blood in the stool, and the child being ill for five days all point toward a bacterial cause.

Question 3 — You should:

A) Ask the mother more questions.

B) Examine the patient further.

C) Order a stool culture, blood tests and intravenous fluids.

D) Call a pediatrician to see the child.

E) All of the above

Answer —

E) is correct.

"Mrs. Meeks, has Ginger eaten any raw clams or oysters?"
"Never."
"Has she been out of the country in the past couple of months?"
"No, she's never been out of the country."
"Any pets at home?"
"A guinea pig. We've had Sparky for two years now. Oh, and the boys got an iguana about a month ago."
"An iguana?" you say.
"Iggy, the iguana. A large, green lizard."
"Has Ginger handled the iguana?"
"Sure, all the kids pick Iggy up."
"The iguana may be the culprit, then. Reptiles, including turtles, snakes, and lizards, often carry *Salmonella* bacteria. The germ doesn't hurt the animal, but little children, especially, are susceptible to *Salmonella* infections. I'll bet Ginger has *Salmonella*."
"Is it treatable, doctor?"
"Very much so. Intravenous fluids will treat her dehydration, and antibiotics can help her body fight the infection. I expect Ginger will perk up pretty quickly."

"I hope so."
"So do I, so do I."

Medical note: Pet reptiles can transmit Salmonella *bacterial infections, some very serious, to humans. Small children are especially susceptible. With reptile pets, persons handling the pets or cleaning the pets' cages should wash their hands thoroughly when done. The kitchen sink should not be used to wash reptiles or their cages.* ❖

SEIZURE

Your patient is: Bernie Doone, a 41 year-old having a seizure.

"Doctor, you're needed in Room 2," the ward clerk says. "A patient is having a seizure."

Seconds later, you slip through the blue curtain into Room 2.

"His seizure has lasted about 60 seconds so far," Nurse Able reports. She wraps oxygen tubing around the patient's head and adjusts it to flow into his nose.

A middle-aged male lies on the stretcher. The torso of his body is rigid. His arms jerk back and forth in a rapid, staccato pattern. His head is twisted to the right. Only the whites of his eyes show. A light froth of saliva surfaces on his lips, while his skin glistens with sweat.

Question 1 — You should:
- A) Force a stick into the patient's mouth to make sure he doesn't bite his tongue.
- B) Give a shot into the patient's arm muscle to stop the seizure.
- C) Apply 400 watt-seconds countershock to the patient's brain to stop the seizure.
- D) Put a breathing tube into the patient to breathe for him.
- E) Wait another minute for the seizure to stop. Protect the patient from hurting himself (keep him from falling off the stretcher).

Answer —
E) is correct. Most seizures last only a few minutes and are not life-threatening. No immediate therapy needs to be given except to protect the patient from harm.

The seizure stops 20 seconds later. The patient begins to take deep breaths, working to restore oxygen to his body.

"Stick an IV line in," you tell Nurse Able. "If he starts to seize again, we'll need to give IV medicine to stop the seizure."

On further examination, the patient appears to be asleep. His pupils are equal and react to light, his reflexes are brisk and equal, his neck supple. There is no sign of an injury to the head.

Question 2 — Your next step is to:
A) Ask the patient questions.
B) Ask the patient's family questions.
C) Examine the patient further.
D) Order a CAT scan (X-ray) of the brain.
E) Call a neurologist (brain specialist) to see the patient.

Answer —
B) is correct. The patient is "post-ictal" (a groggy post-seizure state from which he should slowly awaken over the next 30 minutes). The best source of information is the patient's family.

"I'm Bernie's wife," the short, rotund female says.
"Has your husband had seizures before?"
"He's had them for years, but not very often."
"Has your husband had any fever or infections recently? Has he fallen and hit his head?"
"No."
"Nothing new that might have caused him to have a seizure today?"
"Nothing new. I'll bet Bernie just stopped taking his seizure medicine. He has a habit of taking himself off Dilantin from time to time."
"That may well explain his seizure. We'll check his Dilantin blood level."

An hour later, Nurse Able clips the Dilantin level results to Mr. Doone's chart. *Low, less than 1.0*, it reads.

Back in Room 2, Mr. Doone is sitting up, drinking orange juice.
"How do you feel, Mr. Doone?"

"Pretty good. What happened?"

"You had a seizure at home. You had another one here in the emergency department. Do you remember anything?"

"Just getting a funny taste in my mouth, like I usually do before a seizure."

"Your Dilantin level is low. I guess you've not been taking your medicine?"

Mr. Doone grins sheepishly.

"I guess not, doc. You going to give me some Dilantin through my veins?"

"You bet. We're going to get your level back up to what it should be. Then it'll be up to you."

Mr. Doone tugs on your sleeve.

"Doc, one more thing," he whispers. "I drive a school bus for a living. You won't report this to the authorities, will you?"

"Mr. Doone, if you drive a school bus, you know you should never stop taking seizure medicine unless a doctor tells you to. What do you think would happen if you had a seizure while you're driving?"

"Bad news, I know. I should stay on my medicine."

Question 3 — You should:

A) Inform the patient's mother about the seizure.

B) Tell Mrs. Doone her husband should not drive for at least two hours.

C) Inform the parents of the children riding the school bus.

D) Inform the state driver's license authorities.

E) Inform no one except the patient unless he gives permission.

Answer —

D) is correct. Usually, patient-doctor treatment is privileged information, not divulged to anyone unless permission is given by the patient. In this situation, tragedy and public injury might result if the patient suffers a seizure while driving a school bus. Many states require doctors to report seizures if the patient has a driver's license.

"Mr. Doone," you say, "I am obligated by state law to inform the driver's license authorities that you had a seizure."

"I understand," Mr. Doone replies.

"Also, Mr. Doone, you should not operate a motor vehicle or perform any other hazardous activities until a doctor deems it safe. I will tell your wife the same thing. She needs to know, too. And, please, for goodness sake, stay on your seizure medicine until a doctor tells you to stop."

"OK, doc, I'll stay on my medicine. And I'll go see my neurologist next week to make sure my Dilantin level is in the right range." ❖

BB Boo-Boo

Your patient is: Julie Camacho, 11 years-old.

"It was only a BB gun," Nurse Able says, "but she's complaining of pain in the abdomen."

"Let's go see her," you answer.

The girl lies on her side on the stretcher.

Her mother hovers beside the stretcher, her attention riveted on her daughter. She pushes long, dark hair off her daughter's face, tucking it behind the girl's ear.

"What happened to you, Miss Julie?" you ask.

"I was playing outside on the dirt pile. Juan Valdez was there, too, with his BB gun. He pointed it at me, just playing, but I think he shot me. My stomach began to hurt."

"How is your breathing?"

"Fine."

"Show me where it hurts."

Julie turns over on her back and pulls the hospital gown up to her rib cage, exposing her flat abdomen.

"Right here," she says, pointing to a red circle the size of a BB, just below the bellybutton.

"I need to check your stomach," you say, slipping on a pair of exam gloves.

You press on the girl's abdomen, every place but over the wound.

"Does it hurt when I press?"

"Not really."

Your gloved finger presses right on the wound.

"That hurts!"

The tip of your glove shows a tiny smear of blood.

Question 1 — You should:

A) Tell the police to put out an APB for Juan Valdez.
B) Put a magnet on the wound to suck out the BB.
C) Take X-rays.
D) Numb the wound and probe it with instruments to see if the BB is just under the skin.
E) Tell the mother to watch Julie at home and call you if her daughter vomits or has increasing pain.

Answer —

C) is correct.

"We need to take X-rays to see if a BB is inside you."
Julie bites her lower lip. "OK."
"Can my husband come back?" her mother asks.
"Sure."
Ten minutes later, you flip two X-rays onto the viewbox on the wall.
You point with your index finger to a small, white circle in the center of one film.
"This is the BB," you say. "Metal shows up bright white on X-rays."
The girl and her mother nod. Julie's father, a short, stocky man with a mustache, peers intently at the films.
"The front view shows there is a BB inside you, but it doesn't show whether it's just under the skin or deep inside your body. The side view shows for certain — the BB is four inches inside your abdomen."

Question 2 — You should:

A) Prescribe antibiotics by mouth and let the girl go home.
B) Give intravenous antibiotics and watch the girl in the hospital.
C) Numb the skin and probe the abdomen to remove the BB while the girl is in the emergency department.
D) Order blood tests, a urinalysis, intravenous antibiotics, and call a surgeon.

You Are the ER Doc!

Answer —
D) is correct.

"Your daughter needs an operation," you tell the parents.
"For a BB?" asks the father.
"A BB is a bullet, only smaller. It may have hit a blood vessel or put a hole in the stomach, intestine, liver, or spleen. We won't know until a surgeon looks inside."
Julie's father smashes his fist into the palm of his hand.
"I'll kill that Juan Valdez, I tell you. I'll kill the little punk."
"Hector," his wife says, "Control yourself. Juan Valdez is only 12 years-old. You'll not harm a hair on his body."

Question 3 — By law, you must:
A) Help the father find Juan Valdez and beat him up.
B) Find Juan Valdez and make him watch the surgery.
C) Tell the police to lock up the girl's father until Juan Valdez is in jail.
D) Take no action since Juan Valdez is a minor.
E) Report the BB-gun injury to the police.

Answer —
E) is correct. In most states, an injury involving a firearm must be reported to the police.

One hour later, green scrubsuit-clad surgical technicians roll Julie into the operating room.
After the surgery, the surgeon stops by the emergency department.
"Four holes in the small intestine," she says, shaking her head. "Could have been worse," she adds. "Could have hit the girl's aorta."
"People don't realize how dangerous BB guns are, do they?" you say.
"No, they don't."
"About 25 people in the United States die every year from BB gun injuries. Most of them are children."
"Such a tragedy," answers the surgeon. ❖

Bean in the Nose

Your patient is: Cory Mills, a 2-year-old with a bean up his nose.

Cory sits on his mother's lap. He's a bright-eyed boy with flaxen blond hair.

"I don't know how he got it up there," his mother says. "I try to keep a close watch on him, but you know how two-year-olds are."

The boy's father stands nearby. He crosses his arms on his chest and looks down at the floor. Silently, he shakes his head back and forth.

"This isn't the first case of something-up-the-nose we've had," you reassure the parents.

You slip a Donald Duck finger puppet on your index fingertip and wiggle it in front of the boy's face.

"Hi, Cory."

Cory smiles.

"Can Donald look in your nose?"

Cory nods yes.

"Lie down and put your head on your mom's legs."

Cory cooperates. The Donald Duck puppet directs a light beam from a penlight into Cory's nose. Sure enough, deep inside the boy's right nostril lies a white object.

Question 1 — You should:
A) Tell the parents not to worry, the bean can stay put — but a bean plant may grow out of Cory's nose.
B) Give syrup of ipecac to make the boy vomit.
C) Hold the boy down and pull the object out with a metal instrument.
D) Put the boy to sleep and take the bean out.
E) Teach the mother to give Cory a magic kiss to get the bean out.

Answer —

E) is correct. The bean must come out, or infection may occur. Pulling the bean out with a metal instrument risks injuring the inside of the nose. Giving anesthesia to put a patient to sleep involves the risk of rare but serious side effects (but may be necessary if you can't get the bean out). Being a kind and sensible doctor, you choose magic.

"Dad, can you color with Cory a minute?" you ask the father, handing him a coloring book.

"Sure thing," he says.

You take Cory's mother aside, explaining what you want her to do. Mrs. Mills looks puzzled at first, but nods her head in understanding before you're done.

Back in the room, you position yourself on one side of the stretcher, and give a now-nod to Cory's mother, who stands on the other side of the stretcher, even with Cory's head.

"Cory, I want you to lie down and put your head on the pillow, and I'll give you a magic kiss," his mother says. "I want you to close your eyes and open your mouth a little when Mommy kisses you, OK?"

"OK, Mommy," Cory says. Obediently, he flops back on the stretcher, scrunches his eyes closed, and opens his mouth.

Cory's mother leans over the boy and covers his mouth with hers. She presses her finger on the left side of Cory's nose, closing the left nostril, and blows a puff of air into his mouth.

Cory's mother stands up abruptly. She raises her hand to her face and wipes her cheek.

"Oooh, gross," she says, contemplating the mucus-covered bean in her hand.

"It worked! I blew it out of his nose!" she adds. She laughs, grabs Cory and hugs him tight.

Question 2 — You should:
- A) Tell the boy if he ever puts a bean up his nose again you'll give him a shot.
- B) Tell the parents to give Cory a good spanking when they get him home.
- C) File a report with child protective services since the parents neglected the child and allowed him to get a bean up his nose.
- D) Check Cory's nose again to make sure no other objects are inside, then bid the family adieu.

Answer —

D) is correct.

"Let me shine a light in your nose one more time, Cory."

The light penetrates inside the dark cavern of Cory's nostril. Pink mucous membranes show inside; no bleeding or foreign body is visible.

"Everything looks fine," you reassure the parents. "No more beans up the nose, right Cory?"

Cory nods his head up and down vigorously.

Nice going, doctor, another cure, and a safe one at that. Good trick to remember, the magic kiss treatment. ❖

Bladder Ballast

Your patient is: Marc Inoway, a 25 year-old with a urinary tract problem.

Mr. Inoway sits on the stretcher. He's a thin, young man, cloaked in a faded hospital gown. A brown mustache and wiry, brown hair set off his pale complexion.

The complaint on the chart says, "burning on urination."

"What brings you to the emergency department?" you ask.

"I have another bladder infection. It burns when I urinate, and I have to go all the time."

"*Another* infection?"

"I've had three in the past two months."

"That's highly unusual. Bladder infections are uncommon in males, and three in two months is too many."

Mr. Inoway takes a deep breath and sighs.

"I think I know the reason for the infections," he says.

"What would that be?"

His skin flushes red. He looks down at his feet.

"This is a bit embarrassing, doctor."

"Anything you tell me is confidential information, patient-to-doctor. Nobody else has access to your chart unless you give them permission."

Mr. Inoway closes his eyes and fingers the bridge of his nose.

"I might have something inside of me," he says. "In my bladder."

"What do you think is in there?"

"The inside of a Bic pen. My partner and I got carried away in the heat of passion a couple months ago. My partner put the pen in my penis. We couldn't find the inside piece of the pen afterwards. I think it might be in my body."

"Which would explain the bladder infections. A foreign body acts as a magnet for bacteria."

"I guess so."

On examination, Mr. Inoway's vital signs are normal. He has no pain when a hand is pressed firmly on his lower abdomen. His genitals appear normal. Indeed, his entire exam is normal.

Question 1 — You should:
- A) Call local newspaper and TV reporters to embarrass the patient further.
- B) Call Roto-Rooter.
- C) Tell the patient you don't treat people who do weird sex.
- D) Recommend a psychiatrist.
- E) Order a urinalysis and an X-ray of the lower abdomen.

Answer —
E) is correct.

The urinalysis was already ordered by one of your excellent emergency department nurses. The report reads: *too-numerous-to-count white blood cells, 4+ bacteria* — positive for infection.

The X-ray shows a bright spot, the size and shape of the metal tip of a writing pen, in the area just above the patient's pubic bone. A faint line extends four inches from the bright spot, likely the plastic tube of a pen.

Question 2 — You should:
- A) Tell the patient that he should be able to write with deep inner feelings from now on.
- B) Treat the patient with an antibiotic and send him home.
- C) Treat the patient with an antibiotic in the hospital.
- D) Make immediate preparations to cut into the patient's abdomen and bladder to remove the pen.
- E) Call a urologist.

Answer —
E) is correct. Antibiotics alone will not cure the problem. An object inside the body must be removed if the object is causing infection.

"Mr. Inoway, I'll need to call a urologist to take out the pen. The urologist can do a cystoscopy, putting an instrument through the penis into the bladder, to remove the pen. A cystoscopy has to be done in the operating room, but, if everything goes well, you should be able to go home later the same day."

Mr. Inoway rolls his eyes at the ceiling.

"Oh, this is so embarrassing."

"We've seen objects inside people in all kinds of locations, Mr. Inoway. You're not the first, believe me."

"I've got no choice, do I? It's got to come out."

"Yes, it does. I'll call the urologist. We'll make arrangements to get the pen out."

Hours later, you're finishing the voluminous paperwork of an exhausting ten-hour shift. The urologist pokes his head around the corner of the cubicle where you sit.

"Got the pen out, no problem."

"That's great."

"The nurses in the OR couldn't decide which commercial the patient should audition for," the urologist says, smiling. "They suggested either, *If you can't come, write,* or *Three months in the bladder and it keeps on writing.*"

Throwing your head back, you enjoy a hearty laugh.

Sometimes humor is a great stress equalizer. ❖

Chest Pain

Your patient is: Charles Mann, a 33 year-old man with chest pain.

Mr. Mann lies on the stretcher, his head raised about 30 degrees. A hospital gown covers his thin torso. His skin is pale, and he nervously drums his fingers on his stomach. Clear oxygen tubing snakes into his nose, and an IV line enters his left arm.

"How do you feel right now?" you ask.

"It still aches here." Mr. Mann puts his right hand over his breastbone, in the center of his chest. He sweeps his hand down his left shoulder. "It goes down my arm, too."

"When did it start?"

"About an hour ago, at work. I was outside chopping weeds."

"Any nausea?"

"A little."

"Shortness of breath or sweating?"

"My skin broke out in a sweat when it first came on. My breathing's fine."

"Ever had any heart problems? Treatment for diabetes or high blood pressure?"

"Nope."

"Heart attacks run in your family?"

"Nope."

"Do you smoke?"

Mr. Mann points to his clothes heaped into a pile next to the bed. A pack of cigarettes offers mute evidence, lying half-in, half-out of his shirt pocket. "I'm trying to quit those things, but it's hard."

You Are the ER Doc!

Question 1 — Possible causes of the patient's pain include:
A) Heart attack.
B) Collapsed lung.
C) Gallstones, stomach ulcer.
D) Strain of chest wall muscles.
E) All of the above.

Answer —
E) is correct. Any of these problems (and more) could be causing the patient's chest pain.

Question 2 — Risk factors for heart attack in this patient include:
A) Thin body, nervous habits.
B) Age.
C) Male, smoking.
D) Physically active job.
E) Lack of high blood pressure.

Answer —
C) is correct. Men and smokers are at higher risk for heart attack. Other risk factors, not present in this patient, include age >50, diabetes, high blood pressure, heart attack in the past, and inactive life-style.

You examine Mr. Mann, placing your stethoscope on the front and back of his chest and listening carefully.

"Sounds good," you tell Mr. Mann.

"Here's his heart tracing," Nurse Able says, handing you a sheet of graph paper with squiggles on it.

Normal EKG, reads the computer interpretation at the top. Trusting no machine, you scan the tracing. This time, you agree with the computer: The heart tracing is normal.

Question 3 — You should:
A) Give two aspirin and send the patient home.
B) Give one aspirin and recommend admission to the hospital.
C) Give a shot of Demerol and send the patient home.
D) Throw Mr. Mann's pack of cigarettes on the ground and grind them to shreds under your foot.
E) Get a blood test to tell you if the patient is having a heart attack.

Answer —

B) is correct. You recommend admission because the cause of Mr. Mann's pain is uncertain. Even with a normal heart tracing, he could still be having a heart attack. If a heart attack occurs, the patient's heart could suddenly stop beating. If he is in the hospital, the chances of restarting the heart are much better than if he is at home.

Blood tests do not reliably exclude a heart attack within the first hour after onset of pain.

A single aspirin is given in case Mr. Mann is having a heart attack. Aspirin has been proven to help prevent a heart attack in this situation.

Good job, doctor, you took excellent care of Mr. Mann. Remember, as an emergency medicine doctor, it's your job to think of the worst and hope for the best. In this case, excluding a heart attack is crucial. ❖

Chest Pain/HMO

You are the emergency medicine doctor on duty in the Hometown Hospital Emergency Department, in the middle of a busy shift.

The back of your wrist slides over your forehead, as you wipe away the beads of sweat. You pull the latex gloves off your hands with a snap.

"OK, we can let him out of the papoose," you say.

Nurse Able pulls on the velcro straps holding the cloth papoose in place. The 5 year-old you have just finished sewing up leaps into his mother's arms.

"Thank you, doctor," says the mother. "Tommy, tell the doctor thank-you," she adds.

The boy buries his face in his mother's shoulder, speechless.

"That's all right," you allow. "Nurse Able will go over wound care with you. The stitches need to come out in five to six days. Let me go finish up Tommy's chart and we'll get you going."

But, before you move an inch, Nurse Worthy tugs on your sleeve. "The guy with chest pain, Mr. Mann, says he doesn't want to come in the hospital now," he says. "His wife called their HMO. The HMO rep won't authorize the admission."

Question 1 — You should:

A) Scream louder than the five year-old.

B) Tell the nurse to send Mr. Mann home.

C) Take a dose of antacid to calm your stomach.

D) Call Ask-a-Lawyer for advice.

E) Go talk with the patient, Mr. Mann.

Answer —

    E) is correct.

You stifle the urge to scream, telling the nurse, "I'll go talk to Mr. Mann."

"Mr. Mann," you begin, "I thought we agreed you need to come in the hospital. There's a small chance you're having a heart attack. If so, your heart could stop. If you're at home, there's not much we can do. If you're here, we can treat you."

"Doctor, I understand, but the chances of a heart attack are pretty small, and my wife called our HMO. Hometown Hospital isn't on their preferred provider list, so they won't pay for the admission."

"If I talk to them, will you agree to come in the hospital?"

"If they cover the cost, I will."

Minutes later, the secretary says, "I'm transferring the Healthy Patients HMO representative to your line, doctor."

Nurse Worthy steps to your side as you reach for the phone. "There's an 83 year-old lady coming in by rescue squad with a stroke. They're three minutes out."

You flash an OK sign to Nurse Worthy as you speak into the phone, "Ma'am, I have Mr. Mann here, a 33 year-old male with chest pain, nausea, and sweating. The pain goes down his left arm. He's a smoker. We need to admit him to rule out a heart attack and look for other causes of pain if the heart tests look OK. What's this I hear about you not authorizing the admission?"

"I'm sorry, doctor, but he's pretty young to be having a heart attack, and Hometown Hospital is not on our list of preferred providers. The patient shouldn't have come to your hospital for treatment."

"Let me get this straight. An emergency doctor says a patient needs to come in the hospital for a possible heart attack, and you won't authorize it?"

"My hands are tied, doctor. I have to go by the written protocol here in front of me."

"Can I talk to your supervisor?"

"It's after hours. But I can have her call you in the morning. I

YOU ARE THE ER DOC!

have another suggestion for you, though."

"What's that?"

"Transfer Mr. Mann across town to Westside Hospital. They're on our list of preferred providers."

"You want me to run the risk of Mr. Mann getting worse on the way to the another hospital?"

"I'm afraid that's your only choice if Healthy Patients HMO is going to authorize this admission."

"You mean authorize payment for this admission."

"That's correct."

"Grrrrrr," you say, hanging up the phone.

Nurse Worthy taps on your shoulder. "The stroke patient is in Room 3. She just had a seizure."

Off you dash to Room 3. You do a quick exam of the patient, then scurry back to the nursing station to order multiple blood tests, intravenous medicine to prevent seizures, and a CAT scan of the brain.

"Aargh," you say, glancing at the five charts lined up in the patients-to-be-seen rack. The complaints at the top of the charts read, *cut lip, sore throat, back strain, sprained foot, ingrown toenail.*

Question 2 — What is your next step?

A) Take a dinner break now because your union contract guarantees it.

B) Scream like the five year-old, plus stomp your feet and hold your breath until you turn blue.

C) Tell the nurse the HMO won't pay, to discharge Mr. Mann.

D) Transfer Mr. Mann to the cross-town hospital that accepts Healthy Patients HMO insurance.

E) Go see the five new patients waiting for care.

F) Go talk to Mr. Mann again.

Answer —

F) is correct. Your priorities are excellent, doctor. Mr. Mann has potentially the most serious problem. You hurry to talk with him again, asking the nurse to make sure his wife is in the room.

"Mr. Mann, I feel strongly that you need to be admitted to this hospital at least 24 hours to make sure you're not having a heart attack. Unfortunately, the HMO won't authorize payment to our hospital. The HMO wants me to transfer you to Westside Hospital, but transferring you wouldn't be safe just yet. I think your HMO will eventually come to its senses and pay for your admission here, but I can't guarantee it. I will write letters, call the newspapers, do whatever it takes to get the HMO to pay your bill, though."

"He's decided to come in the hospital," Mrs. Mann says. "We'd rather be safe than sorry."

"A wise decision."

Breathing a sigh of relief, you proceed to take care of the other patients in the emergency department. Mr. Mann is admitted to Hometown Hospital.

Nice job, doctor. You've upheld the doctor's golden rule of always acting in the patient's best interest. Take care of the patient — not the interests of the insurance company or anyone else. ❖

You Are the ER Doc!

Big Bart

You are the emergency medicine doctor on duty in the Hometown Hospital Emergency Department.

The radio crackles to life: "Medic 4 to Hometown Hospital. We're enroute with a comatose male, approximately 30 years old, found in a pickup truck outside his residence. Vital signs are stable. We're five minutes out."

By the time the EMTs push the gurney into Room 3, you and several nurses stand ready.

A large, white male lies on the stretcher. He is clad in faded jeans and a tattered, white t-shirt. His clothes are damp. He breathes steadily. His skin color is normal.

"He's a fisherman, doc," an EMT says. "His name's Grim, Bart Grim. Mr. Grim's family says they found him like this in his truck. He'd been out fishing all day."

Question 1 — You should:
   A) Yell loudly in the patient's ear.
   B) Rub hard with your knuckles on the patient's breastbone.
   C) Press hard on the patient's forehead above his eyeballs.
   D) Give Narcan (narcotic reversal) and D-50 (sugar) intravenously.
   E) Check the patient's blood glucose and blood oxygen level.
   F) All of the above.

Answer —
   F) is correct.

"Narcan, 2 mg, and D-50, 1 amp IV push," you direct. "Check an oxygen saturation and do a fingerstick glucose."

"Bart, wake up!" you yell in the patient's ear. "Wake up!"

Your knuckles dig hard into his breastbone. You pinch the skin on his arm.

Mr. Grim lies still, showing no reaction to your efforts.

You pull up your patient's eyelids. His black pupils are equal in size. Each pupil shrinks in diameter when a bright penlight is shined onto the surface of the eye.

Your fingertips probe the back of Mr. Grim's head and neck. No lumps or cuts are present. The unmistakable odor of stale beer drifts upward from Mr. Grim's face.

"Vitals?" you ask.

"Pulse 88, blood pressure 148 over 86, respirations 18," comes the response. "Oxygen saturation normal at 98%, blood glucose 100, normal."

"Rectal temperature?"

"Normal, 99 degrees even."

"Not hypothermic," you answer. "Get the lab to draw a blood alcohol level, blood count, electrolytes, and drug screen. Order a stat CT scan of the brain."

You turn and walk from the room. Four charts sit in the waiting-to-see-the-doctor rack. *Cough and congestion, cut hand, pus draining from the eyes, might be pregnant,* read the complaints on the charts. You grab the first chart and head for Room 10.

"Lie back down!" comes a cry from Room 3.

"Get the f... out of my way, lady," in response.

Quickly, you detour back to Room 3.

Mr. Grim stands next to the stretcher, wobbly on his feet. He looks down at his right forearm, then yanks the clear, plastic IV tubing out of his arm. He stares as a rivulet of blood flows down his wrist and drips from his hand onto the floor.

Your patient teeters back and forth and falls backward to the floor, landing on his behind.

"Mother f...." he blurts.

"Mr. Grim," you say, "lie back down on the stretcher, please."

"I'm gettin' out'a here," he says, struggling to get to his feet.

"Come on, Mr. Grim, you need help," Nurse Able says. She reaches for his arm, attempting to steady him.

With Able's help, Mr. Grim stands again. Able, still holding his arm, steers him back toward the stretcher.

The patient stops in place. He gazes at Able through glazed, bloodshot eyes. He opens and closes his eyes several times, an apparent attempt to comprehend what he sees.

Suddenly, he lashes out with his log-sized forearm, knocking the nurse to the floor like a child flinging a Raggedy-Ann doll during a tantrum.

"Nobody messes with Big Bart. Get out'a my d... way," he drones.

Question 2 — You should:

A) Tackle Mr. Grim and pin his arms behind his back.

B) Order the nurses to tackle Mr. Grim and restrain him.

C) Shoot Mr. Grim with a sedative gun kept in the emergency department for unruly patients.

D) Contact the hospital's lawyer to ask what is the safest course from a legal viewpoint.

E) Call hospital security personnel and local police to stop Mr. Grim.

Answer —

E) is correct. Your job is taking care of people, not subduing them.

"Back off," you advise your staff. You shoot a glance toward the ward secretary sitting at the central desk. "Ruby, Code Red."

"Already done," comes the answer.

Mr. Grim lurches out of Room 3 like a raging bull. "Get out of my way," he bellows. He staggers toward the glass doors at the ambulance entrance of the emergency department. A trail of red spots marks his progress, blood dripping from his fingers onto the white linoleum floor.

Mr. Grim stops short when he reaches the glass doors. He yells, "Open the f... up," at the doors. He fails to notice the chrome security button on the wall that opens the doors.

"If you won't open up, I'll open you up," he says.

Mr. Grim's foot flies outward at one of the doors, striking it with a thud. On the second try, the door sails forth, jumping out of its tracks and crashing onto the concrete sidewalk outside. The plate glass shatters into a thousand pieces.

Big Bart steps outside, his shoes crunching on the shards of glass. He snorts twice and spits a hunker on the sidewalk. His attention is diverted as two squad cars screech to a halt twenty yards from him.

Four police officers jump from the vehicles and surround Big Bart. He stands still with his hands at his sides, like a deer frozen in the glare of headlights.

One officer pins Big Bart's arms behind him and snaps handcuffs on his wrists.

"What do you want me to do with this fellow, doc?" the officer asks.

> **Question 3** — You should:
> A) Advise the officer, "Book him, Dan-O."
> B) Advise Nurse Able if she would like, she can kick Mr. Grim three times in his rear end.
> C) Tell Mr. Grim he'll have to glue the broken door back together in his spare time.
> D) Inject the patient with a hefty tranquilizer.
> E) Tell the officer to bring Big Bart back into the emergency department so you can finish your evaluation.
>
> **Answer** —
> E) is correct.

"Officer, I need to make sure Mr. Grim is OK health-wise. He's probably just drunk or drugged, but he could have a brain injury. Put him back in Room 3, please."

"I don't want to be checked," Mr. Grim bellows. "Take me to jail. Call my lawyer. I ain't staying here and I ain't paying no emergency room bill."

"What about it doc? He doesn't want to be checked. We can run him in on a disorderly conduct charge."

"I have to check him first. When I'm sure he's OK, you can do whatever you want with him."

"Hey, f... you, doc. I got rights. I'm an American citizen. You lay one hand on me, I'll file charges for assault and battery."

Question 4 — You should:

A) Respect Mr. Grim's wish and not bother him further.

B) Give Mr. Grim an OA (Obnoxious Anonymous) referral and release him.

C) Tell the officer, "Take him downtown."

D) Tell the officer to rap the patient a couple times on the head with a nightstick to get him in line.

E) Evaluate Mr. Grim as planned.

Answer —

E) is correct.

You put your face in front of your patient's face and look him square in the eyes.

"Mr. Grim, you have lost the right to refuse treatment since you were brought here in a coma and are probably intoxicated at present. You are not mentally competent to make a decision for yourself. If I let you go now and you walk out in the street and get run over, unfortunately the courts will hold me responsible. The only right you have in this emergency department is for reasonable and humane treatment, *if* you cooperate."

"Eat it, doc. You can't make me cooperate."

"No, but if you don't, I can legally tie you to the stretcher, put you in a straight jacket, give you a sedative shot, do whatever it takes to control you until I clear you medically. And don't think for a second I won't do these things to keep you still."

"Here's my answer, asshole." Big Bart snorts, then lets fly with another hocker, aimed at your head.

Fortunately, you duck. The policeman behind you is not as quick; a glob of white snot lands on the blue shirt of his uniform.

"Why you no-good son of a —" the officer says, moving toward Big Bart, nightstick in hand.

"Hold it, Rossi," another officer says. "We got other ways of handling bozos like this."

The officer pulls a piece of cloth from his pocket. He ties it securely around Bart Grim's face, pulling it tight through his mouth.

"Mff ffr, dmm fwip," come muffled expletives from behind the gag.

Question 4 — Your options now include:

A) Physically restraining Mr. Grim by tying him to a stretcher with leather restraints.

B) Administering a tranquilizer to calm Mr. Grim.

C) Keeping Mr. Grim under police guard in the emergency department.

D) Letting the officers and Nurse Able take Mr. Grim in a back room and whip some sense into his head.

E) A), B), and C).

Answer —

E) is correct — however tempting D) may be.

As the police lead Big Bart back to Room 3, you order, "Able, draw up 5 mg of Haldol. Have several large people sit on Mr. Grim so he can't budge an inch, then stick the Haldol in his arm. That should calm him a bit."

"Got it, doctor," Able replies.

"After you give the Haldol, tie him to the stretcher with leather restraints. Be careful that someone is with him at all times. He'll need the gag removed and he needs to be turned on his side if he has to vomit, or else he'll suck vomit into his lungs."

"Got it. Hog tie one jerk, but let him loose if he can't breathe or starts to vomit."

"And have lab draw a blood alcohol and a drug screen. See if you can find his family."

"The ward secretary already called the family. They said he's done this several times before and to just send him home by cab when he's ready."

"Have the secretary call the family back and insist they come here now. Tell them I said so. If they were concerned enough about Mr. Grim to call the rescue squad, they can surely come here and help us take care of him."

"Let me know if Mr. Grim changes for the worse," you add. "I've got to go see some other patients."

Three patients and one hour later, you slip back into Room 3.

"Here's one reason for his being so ornery," Able says. She

hands you a white lab slip. *Blood alcohol 424 mg/dl. Drug screen negative*, it reads.

"Ah, yes. A blood alcohol more than five times the legally intoxicated level," you say.

Ten patients and three hours later, you walk back into Room 3 once more.

"Doc, I'm ready to go home," says Mr. Grim.

He sits on the stretcher, sipping Gatorade, his head downcast.

"I'm sorry if I've been a jerk," he adds.

A thin woman, her face prematurely wrinkled, her eyes ringed by dark circles, sits on a stool by the stretcher.

"He gets like this when he drinks," she says. "Normally, he's a good man, a hard worker. When he gets liquor in him, though, there's no telling what he'll do."

"You feel like he's acting normal now?" you query.

"He's hisself, that's clear."

You place your hand on Mr. Grim's shoulder, eye-to-eye once again.

"Mr. Grim, you can go home now. I wish that we had videotaped your performance. Maybe then you would realize what a fool you made of yourself. One of these days, you're going to hurt or kill yourself or someone else because of your drinking. I advise you to never touch a drop of alcohol again as long as you live."

"I'll try, doc, I'll try."

"Alcoholics Anonymous can help if you're willing. Here's a card with their number on it."

Medical note: Treating an alcohol/drug intoxicated patient against his/her will is one of the most challenging situations in emergency medicine. The emergency doctor is "caught between a rock and a hard place." On one hand, following the patient's wishes, and not treating, may result in irreparable harm to the patient. On the other hand, treating the patient is often a thankless, time-consuming, and even hazardous task. Yet, treatment of such patients to the best of one's ability is the course an emergency doctor must follow. ❖

Wormy Meal

Your patient is: Tommy Orlo, a 2 year-old who ate a worm.

"He was sitting outside next to a bush and put this ugly thing in his mouth," his mother says. "A few minutes later, the side of his mouth swelled up, and he started crying."

She holds up a peanut butter jar, empty except for a two-inch, black, worm-shaped animal inside.

The mother hands you the jar. Holding the jar up to your face, you inspect the critter. It's divided into multiple segments, like a roll of pennies. Two tiny legs extend off both sides of each body segment, enabling the animal to crawl slowly around the bottom of the jar.

"Lots of legs. Two per body segment. I think it's a millipede, but I'm not sure," you say.

Question 1 — You should:

A) Yell at the boy for putting something so disgusting in his mouth.

B) Yell at the mother for letting the boy put something so disgusting in his mouth.

C) Yell at the millipede for letting the boy put it into his mouth.

D) Turn the jar upside down, dump the millipede out, and grind it into oblivion with the heel of your shoe.

E) Examine the little boy.

Answer —

E) is correct. And, if you think A) or B) are good choices, you've obviously never had a two year-old!

YOU ARE THE ER DOC!

On examination, the boy's color is good. His breathing appears normal. He smiles and talks to himself as he plays with a set of red and green wooden blocks.

Looking closely at the boy's face, no swelling is visible.

"Open up," you say, holding a penlight in hand, shining it at the boy's mouth.

Tommy opens his mouth. A quick glance inside shows no obvious swelling in the cheek, mouth, or throat. The mucous membrane lining the mouth is a normal pinkish-red throughout.

Putting a stethoscope on the boy's chest, you listen to his lungs. Your ears detect quiet movement of air in and out, no wheezing or other abnormal noises.

Question 2 — You should:
- A) Give the boy a shot of epinephrine just to make sure he doesn't have an allergic reaction.
- B) Tell the mother you're positive there's nothing to worry about.
- C) Tell the mother you're pretty sure the animal is a millipede and harmless, but you need to check a book to make sure.
- D) Let the critter crawl on your arm to see if it can bite.
- E) Let the critter crawl on a nurse's arm to see if it can bite.

Answer —
- C) is correct. Nothing wrong with going back to textbooks when you're not certain about the diagnosis and treatment.

On page 764 of *Wilderness Medicine,* you find that millipedes "differ from centipedes in having two pairs of legs per body segment and in lacking apparatus for injecting venom." The book describes centipedes, close cousins of millipedes, as flattened, having one pair of legs on each body segment, and possessing fangs with venom glands.

The picture of a millipede in *Wilderness Medicine* clearly matches the creepy-crawly in the jar: round, with two pairs of legs per body segment.

"Rest assured, Mrs. Orlo, you have nothing to worry about.

This wormy animal is a harmless millipede. Tommy's mouth may have been irritated from the chemicals in the millipede, but there's no chance of real poisoning. Tommy will be just fine."

"I'm so relieved. I thought it was a poisonous worm of some kind. I'll try to keep him from putting anything in his mouth from now on."

"Kind of hard at his age. If you keep Tommy from chewing on electric cords, poisons, and objects small enough for him to swallow and choke on, you'll be doing a good job as a parent."

"Thank you doctor. Lord knows, I do my best." ❖

To Tube, or not to Tube

Your patient is: Pascal Elder, an 88 year-old male.

Mr. Elder lies on the stretcher, unmoving. His pale, frail frame is covered by a faded hospital gown. He stares straight ahead, his vacant eyes reflecting the white ceiling overhead.

"Mr. Elder," you call loudly. "Mr. Elder!"

No response, you note.

You pinch the skin on the patient's arm.

He doesn't grimace or withdraw his arm.

No response to painful stimuli.

Mr. Elder's breathing is noisy and irregular. A rasping sound grates forth each time he moves air in and out. Periods of long, deep breaths are interspersed with ten-second gaps when he does not breathe at all.

Standing opposite you, on the other side of the stretcher, is Daniel Druse, a fourth-year medical student.

Druse peers intently at Mr. Elder. The contrast is striking: the young man's pink, smooth, clean-shaven face, eyes vigilant, studying the old man's yellow, wrinkled, stubbled face, his eyes void of understanding.

"The patient's lips and fingernails are blue," you remark. "Can you tell me the cause, Mr. Druse?"

Mr. Druse brings his hand up to adjust horn-rimmed glasses on his face, as if the movement will help him focus, help him make sense of what his eyes behold.

"Cyanosis, the patient is breathing inadequately to oxygenate his blood," he answers.

"Correct. Tell me about this patient."

You Are the ER Doc!

"An 88 year-old male from Longterm Nursing Home. This is his third stroke. He's been confined to the nursing home since his second stoke, three years ago. His second stroke left him partially paralyzed on the left side and senile. His right side is paralyzed this time. His breathing is irregular and slow."

You glance at the TV-screen heart monitor. The neon-green blips above the baseline are widely spaced.

"His heart's slowing, too," you remark.

"What should we do?" Druse asks.

"Start with the ABCs, simple as that."

"Airway, breathing, circulation," Druse responds. "His airway is open, but he's not breathing very well."

"Right."

Question 1 — You should:

A) Apply oxygen by mask.

B) Administer a drug through the patient's veins to stimulate breathing.

C) Have the student do mouth-to-mouth breathing.

D) Yell at the patient to breathe better or else you'll put a tube in him to breathe for him.

E) Put a tube in the patient to breathe for him

Answer —

E) is correct. Oxygen will help, but if the patient is not breathing on his own, you must assist his breathing.

"We need to intubate him," you say. "Ready?"

"I've never tubed anyone before."

"Good time to learn. I'll walk you through."

"Can I ask something first?"

"Yes, but make it quick."

"This patient is 88 years-old. This is his third stroke. He was vegetating in a nursing home. Should we really put a breathing tube in?"

"Good question," you reply.

You Are the ER Doc!

Question 2 — You should:
  A) See if the patient can tell you if he really wants to be intubated and put on a breathing machine.
  B) Call the nursing home to see if they have "no-code" papers on the patient.
  C) Call the patient's family to see if they want him intubated.
  D) Make the medical student do mouth-to-mouth breathing until you get a code status.
  E) Intubate the patient.

Answer—
  E) is correct.

"Do you know this patient to be a 'no-code,' Mr. Druse?"
"No."
"Then he's a full code. Tube him. We'll talk later."

Minutes later, you stand with the student at the head of Mr. Elder's bed. The two of you peer into the patient's mouth. Intubation equipment gleams on a tray within hand's reach.

Mr. Elder's tongue is dry and cracked, not moist and glistening like normal. Sour breath wafts forth each time the octogenarian exhales. The odor penetrates the thin mask on your face, causing you to hold your breath.

You guide the student's left hand. He inserts a six-inch long, chrome laryngoscope blade into Mr. Elder's throat. The tongue flops to one side, and the smaller, tongue-like epiglottis, deep in the throat, is lifted out of the way. Two openings in the depth of the throat come into view: The hole on top is the trachea, showing thin, white strips of vocal cord on each side. The hole on the bottom is the wrinkled, red esophagus, the passage from the mouth to the stomach.

You press the endotracheal tube, a flexible conduit 16 inches long and the diameter of a person's thumb, into student Druse's right hand. His hand shakes, but he pushes the clear plastic tube between the patient's vocal cords, into the trachea.

"Got it!" declares the student.

"Good job," you say, patting the student on the back. "We'll put Mr. Elder on a respirator to breathe for him and transfer him to the ICU. Then we'll sit down and talk medical ethics." ❖

Pulling the Plug

Your patient is: Pascal Elder, an 88 year-old male who has had a stroke, causing his breathing to slow.

Daniel Druse, a fourth-year medical student, has just put a breathing tube into the patient. Mr. Druse squeezes a black, flexible bag between his hands. Oxygen flows from the bag, through the breathing tube, into Mr. Elder's lungs.

Mr. Elder's chest rises and falls each time the bag is pumped. Otherwise, he lies still, staring blankly at the ceiling, oblivious to his predicament.

A respiratory therapist wheels a respirator, a metal box-on-wheels, into the room. The respirator is pockmarked with dials and gauges. Tubes, supported by extendible metal arms, protrude from the machine.

"Mr. Druse, bag the patient while the therapist gets the respirator ready," you say. "What settings would you like on the respirator?"

The student shuffles his weight from one foot to another.

"I'm not sure what you mean," he says.

"We have to figure how many breaths per minute the machine should give the patient, and how big each breath should be."

"I don't know."

"Let's figure it out," you say. "How many breaths a minute would the patient normally take on his own, and how big a breath?"

"Maybe 16 to 18 breaths a minute. Each breath about half a liter, 500cc."

"Good estimate. Why don't we set the machine on 18 breaths per minute and, allowing for dead space in the tube, about 650 cc per breath? We'll give Mr. Elder 100% oxygen at first, too."

105

"OK by me," the student says.

"Now," you continue, "you asked why we intubated this patient. He's 88 years-old, suffering his third stroke, and has been in a nursing home the past three years. Should we have let nature take its course, allowing this man to die? Or, should we push on full bore, probably our best hope to return Mr. Elder to the nursing home in a vegetative state?"

"There's no point in pushing on," Druse says. "Is there?"

"Maybe not, in your opinion and mine. But, the wish of the patient matters a great deal. And, in the absence of the patient's opinion, the expectations of the family take priority."

"We don't know what the patient wants, because he can't speak. The family's not here. So we don't know what they want."

"Exactly. Maybe the patient himself doesn't want extraordinary measures. Maybe the family doesn't want any heroics. The fact of the matter, though, is that we don't know."

"So we have to assume he wants all the treatments we can offer."

"That's right."

"Doctor, excuse me," a nurse says, poking his face around the curtain. "A family member is here. The patient's daughter."

"Send her in."

A tanned, blond woman, about 60 years old, enters the room minutes later. She steps to the bedside and places her hand on Mr. Elder's forehead.

"Pop, how are you doing?" she asks. Mr. Elder shows no response.

"He's had another stroke?" she asks. A tear rolls down her cheek.

"Yes, a big one. It affected the respiratory center in the brain. We had to put a breathing tube in to help him breathe."

"I wish you hadn't done that," she says. "My father signed a living will. He doesn't want to be kept alive on a breathing machine, especially if he is not with it mentally."

"I'm sorry, we didn't know his wishes," you say. "Do you have the living will with you?"

The daughter hands you a yellow sheet of paper. It's an original record, signed and notarized.

> *I, Pascal Elder, being of sound mind, hereby declare my desire that my life not be prolonged by aggressive medical care unless there is a good chance such measures would be temporary in nature and I would be restored to a useful and productive state....*

"This document is clear," you state. "Is this what you want, too, no breathing tube or respirator?"

"Yes."

"You understand your father will likely die without the machine assisting his breathing?"

The daughter looks at her father. Tears well up in her eyes. She swallows hard.

"I understand," she says. "It's what Daddy wanted and I think it's for the best, too."

Question 1 — You should:
- A) Disconnect the respirator and remove the breathing tube.
- B) Have the hospital lawyer read over the patient's living will before disconnecting anything.
- C) Make the daughter sign a paper promising that she won't sue if you disconnect the respirator and her father dies.
- D) Present the case to the hospital's ethics committee before you disconnect anything.
- E) Leave the tube in place and the respirator working.

Answer —

A controversial question, but A) is probably the best answer.

You press the power button of the respirator with your index finger. The repetitive hiss of air being pushed into the patient's lungs ceases. You unwrap the tape holding the breathing tube to Mr. Elder's face and slide the tube out.

"I have no idea how long he will continue to breathe on his own," you tell the daughter. "Will you stay with him?"

"I'd like to."

You motion to medical student Druse to follow you. The two of you slip out of the room and walk back to the nursing station.

"Can you just pull the plug and take the tube out like that?"

"I just did, didn't I?"

"Yeah, but is it legal?"

"Sure, and ethical, too. It's what the patient wanted, his family wanted, and what we thought was best, too."

"There's no way I want to be a vegetable in a nursing home."

"Most everyone in medicine feels the same way, Mr. Druse. There's a time to live and a time to die for all of us."

Medical note: The importance of planning to facilitate death with dignity can not be stressed enough. Careful discussion with family members prior to medical debility is essential. Legal documents, such as a living will and a health care power of attorney, help insure a person's wishes for end-of-life care are fulfilled. ❖

Surprise Package

You are the emergency medicine doctor on duty in the Hometown Hospital Emergency Department.

With a flick of your wrist, the slender, chrome needle holder in your hand rotates like a screwdriver. The metal needle clamped in the end of the instrument goes into the skin on one side of the wound and out the skin on the other side. Mechanically, the same as thousands of times before, you tie five knots in the black thread attached to the needle. The tightened suture pulls the edges of the wound together.

The reverie of wound suturing is broken by Nurse Able tapping on your shoulder.

"Doctor, I think you need to see the patient in Room 8," she says.

You glance at Able, then back at the three-inch gash on the patient's forearm. The cut is half way closed with spider-like, black stitches.

"What's the patient's chief complaint?" you ask.

"She's a 22 year-old female, complaining of abdominal pain, in the lower part of her abdomen. A cramping type pain that seems to come in cycles about three to four minutes apart."

"Pregnant?" you ask.

"She denies it," Able replies, "Says she hasn't missed a period and has not been sexually active."

"Should we send a urine pregnancy test?"

"I don't think so. Go see what you think."

You Are the ER Doc!

Question 1 — You should:
A) Finish sewing the cut, then go see the patient with abdominal pain.
B) Listen to Nurse Able and go check the patient with abdominal pain now.
C) Ask Nurse Able to call in another doctor to check the patient with abdominal pain.
D) Stand up, stomp your feet, and declare, "I can't be two places at once!"
E) Reprimand Nurse Able for bothering you while you are sewing up a patient.

Answer —
B) is correct. Pay heed to your nurses.

"Mr. Grandy," you say, "I've got to go see another patient, urgently. I'll be back to finish your cut as soon as I can."

"I understand, doctor," he replies.

Standing up, you strip the thin, latex gloves from your hands, flip the plastic face shield off your face, and wiggle out of the yellow hospital gown.

Seconds later, you follow Nurse Able into Room 8. A glance at the chart in your hand reveals that your new patient's name is Wanda White.

Ms. White lies on the stretcher. Her face is red, her lips pursed, and her eyes scrunched shut.

"Where are you hurting?" you ask.

"Down low," she gasps.

You put your hand on Ms. White's abdomen. The muscles are tense in spasm, but they suddenly relax. Ms. White exhales.

"That's better," she says. "The pain comes and goes."

Ms. White's abdomen is large. She is decidedly overweight.

"Here's the doppler. Take a listen for heart tones," Able says.

Nurse Able hands you a small, transistor radio-like box. A microphone is attached to the box by a thin wire.

Able squirts blue-tinged K-Y jelly onto Ms. White's swollen, white abdomen. Holding the microphone in your fingers like a pencil, you slide it slowly back and forth over Ms. White's belly, following the line of jelly.

Harsh static sounds forth from the doppler. Then, a strong, repetitive, woosh, woosh, woosh, replaces the static. The rhythm of the wooshes matches the throbbing pulse your fingers feel on Ms. White's wrist.

Her heartbeat, you think.

You slide the microphone farther to the right. A rapid, *swoosh, swoosh, swoosh, swoosh,* much faster than Ms. White's pulse, sounds forth.

You count the number of swooshes in 15 seconds.

Forty times four, you think, *160 per minute. Good heart rate.*

Question 2 — You should:
  A) Send a urine pregnancy test.
  B) Send a more accurate blood pregnancy test.
  C) Send a urinalysis, blood count, blood type, and pregnancy test.
  D) Time Ms. White's contractions. Do a quick finger check in Ms. White's vagina to see if you can feel the baby.
  E) Ask Ms. White if she has had any contact with aliens.

Answer —
  D) is correct. No need to send a pregnancy test. The baby's heart tones are proof of pregnancy. The pressing question is — how soon is the baby coming?

"Able, are you timing contractions?"
"Three minutes apart."
"Let me have a sterile glove, please."
"Ms. White, I need to do a quick check in your vagina to find out how close the baby is to being born."
"The baby?"
"Yes, baby. You're pregnant."
"Can't be."
"I'm afraid there is no doubt about it."
Ms. White shuts her eyes and bites her lower lip.
You pull a sterile glove onto your right hand. Able squirts sterile K-Y jelly onto your gloved fingers.
"Ms. White, I don't mean to rush you, but time is of the essence. Relax your legs and let them fall apart at the knees."

A tear rolls down Ms. White's cheek, but she loosens her legs. You slide index and middle fingers inside Ms. White's vagina. Your fingers touch a firm object, the size and shape of a cantaloupe.

Question 3 — You should:
   A) Tell Ms. White to cross her legs, keep them tightly closed, and hold her breath.
   B) Pull a white handkerchief out of your pocket. Mop your brow. Yell, "Bring me hot water, a basin, and towels."
   C) Get Ms. White's signed permission to deliver the baby.
   D) Transfer Ms. White to the OB hospital across town for delivery.
   E) Prepare for delivery, immediately.

Answer —
   E) is correct.

"Able, let's set up to deliver. I'll need a gown, face shield, and delivery kit.

"Ms. White, you're about to have a baby. Tell me when your last normal period was."

"How can I be pregnant?" she answers. "I only had sex a couple times last September. I've had periods since then, even though they've been light."

"Intercourse even once can get you pregnant. Your last normal period was September?"

"Right."

"Good. That puts us about nine months. Good chance you'll have a mature baby instead of a preemie."

"The pain's coming again," Ms. White says. Her eyes close and she purses her lips.

"I feel like I need to push with my bottom," she says.

"Just pant, and don't push until the next pain comes."

On the next contraction, you're ready: gowned, gloved, a tray of sterile instruments at hand.

"Oh, my God, it hurts!" cries Ms. White. She holds her breath and pushes.

The baby's head slides out of her vagina.

Question 4 — You should:
   A) Pull the baby out, hold it upside down by the feet, and spank the baby's bottom to make it cry and breathe.
   B) Call for a nurse midwife to come quickly and deliver the baby.
   C) Ask the mother to name the baby after you, since you are delivering her child.
   D) Suction mucus from the baby's mouth.
   E) Use one hand to cradle the baby's neck between your thumb and index finger, and use your other hand for support underneath the baby's body.
   F) When the baby is out, dry it off and wrap it in a blanket.
   G) A), B), and C) are correct.
   H) D), E), and F) are correct.

Answer —
   H) is correct. Clear the baby's airway so it can breathe. Make sure you don't drop the baby. Keep the infant warm.

"A healthy baby girl," you announce as the rest of the child enters the world.

The baby's skin is dusky at first, but pinks up as the baby cries heartily. You listen to the baby's heart with your stethoscope.

"160 and regular, sounds good."

Question 5 — You should:
   A) Clamp the baby's umbilical cord in two places, then cut the cord between the clamps.
   B) Put drops in the baby's eyes as a preventive measure against gonorrhea infection.
   C) Let the baby bond with the mother.
   D) Admit the mother and the baby to the hospital.
   E) Get an ob-gyn doctor to care for the mother, a pediatrician/family doctor to take care of the child, and a counselor/social worker to assist the mother.
   F) All of the above.

Answer —
>   F) is correct. Ms. White and her baby need full physical evaluation and treatment, especially since they had no prenatal (pre-birth) care. In addition, the mother needs psychological and social counseling for this abrupt change in her life.

"Ms. White, I'm clamping the baby's cord and then cutting it. Your body will expel the placenta in a little while. Nurse Able is putting drops in your baby's eyes to prevent infection.

"As soon as I wrap your baby in a warm towel, you can hold her."

You gently place the towel-swathed infant on the mother's chest. Human nature takes over. Ms. White beams at her baby.

"She's beautiful, isn't she!"

"Yes, she is," Able says.

"Beautiful and healthy," you add.

You pause to remove your face shield, gloves, and gown once again. Placing a hand on Ms. White's shoulder, you continue, "You and your baby need to come in the hospital for a day or two. An ob-gyn doctor and pediatrician will take care of the two of you. I would also recommend counseling and visits from our social workers. Having a child means a huge change in your life."

"All right," Ms. White answers. Her smile suddenly disappears. "Nobody will try to take my baby away, will they?"

"Not as long as you're willing to be a good mother," you answer.

"Oh, I'll be a good mother. How could I not be with this bundle of joy?" Ms. White fixes on her infant again with a motherly gaze. ❖

The Alcoholic

Your patient is: Texas Jones, a 53 year-old male.

"The paramedics brought in Texas Jones again, doctor," Nurse Able reports. "He's in Room 5, sound asleep. You want us to send a blood alcohol level?"

She hands you his chart. The paramedics' report reads:
Called to scene when patient found beside Kwik Mart, passed out. Vomit on his shirt. Won't wake up. Smells strongly of alcohol. Picked up with same problem last week.

Question 1 — You should:
A) Call the sheriff's department. Ask law enforcement officers to take Mr. Jones to jail and let him sleep it off there.
B) Transfer Mr. Jones to the county hospital across town.
C) Tell the nurse to let Mr. Jones sleep it off, and to send a blood alcohol level.
D) Tell the nurse to let Mr. Jones sleep it off, but not send a blood alcohol level.
E) Go examine the patient.

Answer —
E) is correct.

"Let's go check ol' Texas," you say, ever the diligent doctor.
The smell streams up your nostrils and assails your brain as soon as you stride into the room. The malodorous mixture of stale alcohol, vomit, body odor, and street dirt is overwhelming.

You Are the ER Doc!

You hold your breath long enough to tie a mask over your mouth and nose. You also don a pair of thin, latex gloves.

The smell still filters through the mask, slowed but not eradicated by the paper barrier.

"Vital signs?" you ask.

"Stable except for a blood pressure of 180 over 110," Nurse Able says. "Not unusual for Mr. Jones. He's a chronic dirigible, and doesn't take care of himself. How can people live like that?"

"I don't know," you answer.

"Mr. Jones, Mr. Jones," you yell in the patient's face. No response.

Your knuckles dig into Mr. Jones's breastbone, rubbing hard. You pinch his arms with your fingertips. No response.

A bright penlight shined into Mr. Jones's eyes reveals large, black pupils. The pupils shrink in response to the beam of light.

"Pupils react normally," you remark.

Your gloved fingers track up the back of Mr. Jones's neck, then through the hair on his scalp. A smear of blood shows on the glove on your left hand. Tracing backwards, your fingertips outline a lump on the side of the skull about the size of half an orange. Lifting strands of greasy, gray hair over the swelling exposes a scrape wound on the skin. Blood oozes from the wound.

Question 2 — You should:

A) Tell the nurse to let you know when Mr. Jones wakes up.

B) Put a tube into Mr. Jones's stomach. Give coffee through the tube to sober up Mr. Jones.

C) Order intravenous caffeine to sober up Mr. Jones.

D) Check an alcohol level to make sure Mr. Jones is just drunk.

E) Order a CAT scan of the brain, blood alcohol level, and other blood tests.

Answer —

E) is correct.

"Texas may be just snockered again," you say, "but I don't like what I see. He could have fallen, or somebody could've whacked him on the head. Let's get a CT of the brain to rule out brain injury, a stat blood sugar since alcoholics can get a low blood sugar, a blood alcohol level, and drug screen."

"Want me to move him to a front room?" Nurse Able says.

"You bet. We need to keep a close eye on Texas until we know what's going on."

Half an hour later, the X-ray tech flips four sheets of black-and-white film images up on the X-ray view box.

"Better take a look at these, doctor," the tech says.

"Uh-oh," you say, scanning the films.

"What's up?" says Nurse Able, standing behind you.

Your index finger traces a shadow on the film.

"See this dark space, shaped like a sliver of moon, right here between the skull and the brain? That's a subdural hematoma, a collection of blood from a broken vein."

"What now?"

"Call neurosurgery, stat. Got to open the skull and suck out that blood."

"What's the prognosis?"

"Not great, especially with Mr. Jones's alcoholism. It makes him at risk for complications. Infection, bleeding, anesthesia reaction, slow recovery, you name it."

"Too late for him to reform now."

"Hopefully, he'll get a chance to reform in the future. He's got to make it through this problem first, though."

Excellent care, doctor. You've given Mr. Jones the highest chance of recovery possible. If you had simply waited for him to wake up, his outcome would be much worse.

Remember: 1) Always examine the patient, and 2) When making a list of possible diagnoses, think of the worst but hope for the best. ❖

Belly Buster

Your patient is: Milo Sills, an 8 year-old with abdominal cramping.

"I thought it was a stomach virus at first, but it doesn't seem to be getting better," says Milo's mother. "So, I brought him in."

Milo's mother brushes the boy's brown hair off his forehead.

"He started vomiting about midnight," she continues. "Then he had a couple episodes of diarrhea about 5 A.M. His pain is getting worse."

Milo lies on his right side on the stretcher, motionless. A *just-don't-feel-good* look masks his face.

"How are you doing, Milo?" you ask.

"Not good," he manages.

"Where does it hurt?"

He points to his abdomen.

"Can you lie flat on your back and point to where it hurts the most?"

Milo rolls over on his back. He points just below his bellybutton.

Your press on the left side of his abdomen, on the top and bottom. Milo doesn't grimace, nor does he cry out in pain.

You press on the right upper abdomen.

"Does that hurt?"

Milo nods his head, yes, but he doesn't flinch.

You press on his right lower abdomen.

Milo draws his legs up and squirms. "Ow!" he says, his face tightening.

"That's where it hurts the most, Milo?"

Milo nods yes.

You Are the ER Doc!

Question 1 — You should:
- A) Check Milo's temperature.
- B) Order a urinalysis.
- C) Order a white blood count.
- D) Order X-rays of the abdomen.
- E) Order a CAT scan of the abdomen.
- F) A), B), and C).

Answer —

F) is correct. Simple tests may suffice to make the diagnosis. X-rays are not needed at this time.

"Milo, we need to do a blood test on you. Drawing the blood will feel like a small bee sting on your arm. OK?"

"OK," answers Milo.

"He's had his blood drawn before," his mother says. "He'll be brave."

Nurse Able sticks a thermometer under the boy's tongue. "Checking again to see if you have a fever, Mr. Milo," she says. The digital readout flashes on the instrument, 100.5°.

An hour later, Milo's lab tests are back: The urinalysis is normal. The boy's white blood count is increased to 15,400 (normal 5,000 to 12,000).

Question 2 — You should:
- A) Advise Milo's mother that Milo has a stomach virus and she can take him home.
- B) Advise Milo's mother to take Milo home and give him only liquids, no solids, until he is better.
- C) Call a surgical doctor and send Milo to the doctor's office.
- D) Call a surgical doctor and recommend Milo be observed in the hospital.
- E) Call a surgical doctor and recommend Milo be operated on soon.

Answer —

E) is correct. *Now* is the time for action.

"Mrs. Sills, we need to get a surgeon here to see Milo promptly. Milo may have appendicitis. The key with appendicitis is not to miss the diagnosis and allow the condition to worsen.

Question 3 — The reason to be careful not to miss appendicitis is:
A) The pain will continue and become increasingly severe.
B) The intestine may rupture (break open).
C) Vomiting may become so severe that it causes internal (intestinal) bleeding.
D) Locked bowel syndrome (severe constipation) may develop.
E) A doctor can be sued for malpractice if he/she doesn't make the right diagnosis every time.

Answer —
B) is correct.

"Mrs. Sills, Milo needs an operation to prevent a complication of appendicitis which can be life-threatening. An inflamed appendix can rupture, spilling feces and intestinal bacteria into the whole abdomen. An abscess or whole body infection can result. The infection can cause severe illness and sometimes even death."

"I surely don't want that to happen," Mrs. Sills says. "But, is this appendicitis for sure, or could Milo have something else?"

"Milo could have an intestinal virus or several other conditions causing his symptoms. But he has enough symptoms to assume he has a hot appendix and take him to the operating room. The risk of anesthesia and surgery is small but real. But, again, if we miss the diagnosis, the results can be disastrous."

"I understand," Mrs. Sills replies. "One more question. What's the function of the appendix? What does it do?"

"The appendix is a worm-like pouch extending off the large bowel. It's a vestigial organ possessed only by humans, apes, and wombats."

You smile and continue, "In simpler terms, nobody knows what the appendix does, but nobody misses it if it's taken out."

"Let's get Milo's vestigial organ or whatever out before it ruptures."

"Right. I'll call the surgeon pronto."

Medical note: The diagnosis of appendicitis is difficult at times. Rarely do patients present with "classic textbook" signs: low fever, vomiting, and abdominal pain starting as mild discomfort in the middle abdomen and shifting to and becoming more intense in the right lower abdomen.

Other signs and symptoms can mask the diagnosis of appendicitis. Diarrhea can occur if the inflamed appendix lies next to the bowel. White blood cells in the urine occur if the inflamed appendix lies near the ureter (the tube from the kidney to the bladder).

Bottom line: The emergency doctor must be careful and diligent in order to detect both obvious and subtle cases of appendicitis. ❖

Intubation Practice

You are the emergency medicine doctor on duty in the Hometown Hospital Emergency Department.

The radio in the emergency department crackles to life.
"Medic-7 to Hometown Hospital."
"Go ahead, Medic-7."
"We have a 76 year-old male in full cardiac arrest. CPR in progress. The heart monitor shows asystole, flatline. We've intubated the patient, given epinephrine and atropine, shocked with 400 watt-seconds, all with no response. This gentleman has a history of two heart attacks in the past."
"How long has the patient been down?"
"Eight minutes till we arrived on the scene, another 20 on scene, 15 minutes enroute. A total of 40 to 45 minutes."
"What's your ETA?"
"We'll be at your back door in three minutes."
The ambulance glides to a stop at the back door, lights flashing. The paramedics hop out and extract the gurney from the back of the vehicle. The medics sidestep next to the stretcher, continuing CPR, as they roll into the emergency department.
On the stretcher is a large, rotund, white-skinned male. The only clothing on the patient is a pair of green, paisley boxer shorts.
The medics bring the patient to Room 1, the "code" room, where you and the nurses stand waiting.
"Do we have a name?" you ask.
"Cease. Samuel Cease. He's been down 50 minutes so far," a paramedic answers.
"On three," says one of the paramedics. "Ready, one, two, three."

Multiple sets of hands grasp the sheet under the patient and lift him over to the hospital's stretcher in Room 1.

Mr. Cease is blue from the nipples up. An IV bag hangs above him, the plastic tubing running into his arm. A breathing tube protrudes from his mouth; his chest rises and falls as a bag connected to the tube is squeezed, pushing oxygen into his lungs.

"Hold up on CPR," you direct.

Feeling for a pulse, your fingers probe Mr. Cease's neck. Your eyes focus on the heart monitor connected to him; the screen shows an electric, green flatline. Your fingertips detect not a hint of blood flowing in his arteries.

"Resume CPR," you state.

A technician resumes her rhythmic pumping on the patient's chest.

You listen with a stethoscope on Mr. Cease's chest. Air moves in when the bag is squeezed: The tube is in place. You shine light into his eyes: The pupils are large and fixed in position — they do not constrict to light.

Question 1 — You should:

   A) Give more epinephrine and atropine (drugs) intravenously.
   B) Administer a shock to the heart.
   C) Start New CPR (alternating pumping on the stomach and chest).
   D) Call a cardiologist.
   E) Call off the code (stop resuscitative efforts).

Answer —

   E) is the only reasonable choice — although some doctors might continue efforts. The chance of successful resuscitation in this situation is zero. The likelihood of returning the patient to a semblance of normal life is nil. Continuing efforts might just prolong Mr. Cease's death, possibly at significant expense and mental anguish to his family.

"Stop all efforts," you direct.

Nurses, respiratory therapists, medical students, and technicians stop the tasks they are performing at the bedside. They file from the room. Quiet ensues.

You check the patient again for pulses, placing your fingertips in the neck and groin. No pulsations are present. Listening with a stethoscope over the chest, no heart sounds are audible. Bright light shined in the patient's eyes reveals large, black pupils, fixed in position.

Your head hangs low.

"I'll be filling out the chart and death certificate," you tell the nurse remaining in the room. "When all the family is gathered, let me know so I can talk to them."

"Sure, doctor," she replies.

The only other person in the room, a tall, young woman wearing a white lab coat, clears her throat.

"Um, excuse me, doctor. Can I practice intubation?" she says. The name tag on her coat reads, *M. Lerner, Medical Student*.

Question 2 — You should:
  A) Never allow a medical student to practice a procedure on a patient: Medical students are not yet doctors.
  B) Allow the medical student to practice intubation on the dead patient while you fill out forms at the nurses' station.
  C) Allow the medical student to practice intubation on the dead patient, supervised by you.
  D) Allow the medical student to practice intubation on the dead patient only if the family gives permission.

Answer —
  A) and B) are incorrect. Medical students need to learn medical skills, but they should be supervised when performing important duties. Choosing between answers C) and D) is difficult. Ethically, getting permission from the family to practice intubation is optimal. Practically speaking, time may not allow gaining consent.

"Put on a pair of gloves," you say. "We'll run through a couple of intubations while we have the chance. Practicing on a corpse may save someone else's life someday." ❖

BRAVE WITH KNIVES, SCARED OF NEEDLES

Your patient is: Hannibal Slocum, a 30 year-old male with cuts on his arm and chest.

Mr. Slocum lies on the stretcher, his hands behind his head, an expansive grin on his face.

"About time, doc," he says.

"I had to see a patient with a heart attack first," you explain.

"That's OK, I was taking a catnap till you got here."

"The chart says you fell on some glass and cut yourself last night."

"That's right," Mr. Slocum replies.

"How come you didn't come in until now, twelve hours later?"

"To tell you the truth, doc, I was drinking."

"Drinking too much these days?" you ask.

"Naw, I can handle it. But I can't handle needles. Doc, you got to promise not to sew on me. Just put a bandage on my cuts."

"Let's take a look at your wounds," you counter.

Mr. Slocum points to the inside of his left arm, half way between his shoulder and elbow. A two-inch cut gapes open. Yellow globs of fat, normally hidden in the tissue layer under the skin, bulge from the cut.

Opposite the arm wound, on Mr. Slocum's chest, is a one-inch cut. The edges of this wound, too, are pulled apart like the lips of an open mouth. Red and yellow tissue lies inside.

"These cuts need to be sewn up, Mr. Slocum," you say. "Number one, they'll heal quicker with sutures. Number two, if we numb the wounds, we can clean them out much better. It won't hurt when we scrub the wounds. And, number three, we can inspect the wounds and make sure no pieces of glass are inside."

"Just the same, doc, I don't want stitches. It'll still heal up if we don't use stitches, won't it?"

"The cuts will heal, Mr. Slocum. But, your wounds will take a *long* time to heal if they aren't closed with sutures."

Question 1 — You should recommend:

A) Suturing the wounds.

B) Mr. Slocum seek a second opinion from another doctor.

C) Mr. Slocum seek a second opinion from his personal advisor.

D) Mr. Slocum go home and think about what he wants and come back tomorrow if he wants sutures.

E) Mr. Slocum chooses whatever treatment he wants.

Answer —

A) is correct. Stick to your guns, doctor. Recommend what you think is the best treatment for your patient.

"Mr. Slocum, my advice is that we sew up your cuts. I'm worried there might be pieces of glass in the wounds."

"Don't worry about that, doc. I'm sure there's no glass inside. See, just between you and me — strictly off the record — I got cut by somebody with a knife last night. That's how I know there's no glass in the wounds."

Question 2 — You should:

A) Ignore what the patient said, since it's "off the record."

B) Ignore what the patient said, since it is privileged patient-doctor information.

C) Tell the patient he should be ashamed of himself for making up a story about how he got cut.

D) Threaten to tell the patient's mother if he doesn't let you sew him up.

E) Threaten to tell the police if he doesn't let you sew him up.

F) Re-examine the patient.

Answer—
F) is correct. Wounds from a knife are potentially much more serious than cuts caused by falling on glass. Re-examine the patient!

You pull a black stethoscope from the pocket of your white coat.
"Take some deep breaths, Mr. Slocum."
The stethoscope slides back and forth, left to right, on the patient's chest.
"Your lungs sound good."
"Now breathe nice and easy." You listen on the left side of the chest, over the heart.
"Your heart sounds fine, too," you state. "But we need to look inside those wounds, especially the one on the chest. It's impossible to tell how deep the wound is just by looking at it. The wounds should be probed to make sure the knife didn't go in deep and injure the heart or lungs."
"Naw, doc, I'm sure the knife didn't go in far. Just put some bandages on the wounds, and I'll be on my way."

Question 3—You should:
A) Consult your crystal ball to see what to do next.
B) Call Ask-a-Lawyer to find out what to do next.
C) Hold Mr. Slocum down and suture the wounds whether he wants it or not.
D) Give Mr. Slocum a knock-out drug and then suture the wounds.
E) Let the patient decide what treatment he wants.

Answer—
E) is correct. Your patient is an adult, capable of making his own decisions. Although he was drinking last night, he is not intoxicated at present and is mentally competent to decide his own fate.

"Mr. Slocum, I'll have the nurse clean the wounds with peroxide and put a bandage on. You need to do the same thing at home once a day. If infection sets in, come right back. And, you should think about stopping drinking. Seems like alcohol might be getting you in trouble."

"Like I said, doc, I can handle my liquor."

"Maybe, maybe not. The next time you might not be so lucky. You might be facing a lot of needles. Think about it!"

"I hear you, doc." ❖

Hip Fracture?

Your patient is: Addie Simmons, an 87 year-old female with hip pain.

Mrs. Simmons is gray-haired and thin, lying on the stretcher with her eyes closed as you enter the room.

She opens her eyes and scrutinizes you with a bird-like countenance.

"It's about time you got here, doctor. I've been waiting almost an hour."

"I apologize, Mrs. Simmons. I was busy with some very sick patients," you answer. "But, I'm here now. Tell me where you hurt."

"It doesn't," Mrs. Simmons answers tartly.

"Did you fall?"

"Haven't even had my dinner," the old lady voices.

Her daughter, sitting on a stool next to the bed, folds one of the old lady's hands in both of hers.

"The rest home staff told me they found Mother on the floor next to her bed. She must have fallen when she got up this morning. She seemed to be okay at first, but the staff said she had pain in the hip off and on all day. The nurse's aide finally called me about four-o'clock this afternoon. I brought Mother right in."

"Has she complained of anything to you?"

"She doesn't complain when she lies still, but if you try to move her she says it hurts in her left hip."

"Feisty, isn't she?" you ask.

"That she is, doctor, that she is."

You Are the ER Doc!

Question 1 — You should:
A) Tell the old lady no line dancing for two weeks.
B) Tell the daughter to give her mother two aspirin and call you in the morning.
C) Make the patient an appointment with an orthopedic (bone) doctor tomorrow.
D) Order an X-ray of the left hip.
E) Examine the patient.

Answer —
E) is correct. Being a competent doctor, you examine the patient before ordering an X-ray.

"That hurts, doctor!" Ms. Addie says when you press on the left hip. She voices no complaint, nor does she grimace, when you press elsewhere on her pelvis, back and legs.

"Left hip X-ray?" asks Nurse Able.

"Yes, indeed," you answer.

"Ms. Addie, I'll be back to see you after your X-rays are done. I need to scoot and take care of some other folks right now."

"I'm not waiting another hour, I'll tell you that," the old lady says.

Twenty minutes and two patients later, the X-ray technician slaps black celluloid films up on the lighted view box.

"There you are, doc."

Carefully, you inspect the X-rays. No sign of a break in the femur, the big bone in the upper leg that forms the ball of the ball-and-socket hip joint. No dislocation of the joint, either.

"Is the radiologist still here?" you ask the X-ray tech.

"Yeah, right," comes the answer.

The clock on the wall reads 6:03 P.M. No, there'll be no help in reading the films tonight. You're on your own.

Question 2 — You should:
A) Tell the old lady to quit complaining, there's nothing wrong.
B) Tell the daughter you think her mother is faking injury to get attention.
C) Tell the daughter to give her mother two aspirin and call the radiologist in the morning.
D) Give the patient a cortisone shot in her left hip.
E) Re-examine the patient.

Answer —

 E) is correct. A fine and caring doctor you are, examining the patient again.

"Ms. Addie, we're going to stand you up and see how you do." "Take her arm on the other side, I've got this side," you tell Nurse Able.

The old lady slides her backside down the side of the bed and lands gently on her two feet. "Ow, ow, ow, my leg," she says, pulling her left leg up off the floor. She is unable to bear weight on the leg, much less walk.

"OK, back to bed, Ms. Addie." You and the nurse lift the patient back into bed.

Question 3 — You should:
- A) Put the patient on crutches and send her back to the rest home.
- B) Prescribe a motorized bed for the patient to get around the rest home until she can walk.
- C) Tell the daughter to give two aspirin and call her mother's regular doctor in the morning.
- D) Put a cast on the old lady from the bellybutton to the knees.
- E) Put the patient in the hospital overnight and schedule an MRI in the morning.

Answer —

 E) is correct. Being a wise and caring doctor, you treat the patient, not the X-ray. The patient has at least a bruised hip, but she could also have a break in the hip that doesn't show up on the X-ray. An MRI will show if there is a hidden fracture. You put Ms. Addie in the hospital until the MRI can be done.

Two weeks later, you get a report from Ms. Addie's hospitalization. The MRI showed a crack in the femur. Surgery was necessary to fix the break.

Way to go, doctor. Always remember to treat the patient, not the X-ray — or blood test, or paper with numbers on it. ❖

Bitten in Person

Your patient is: Taquisha Jones, a 21 year-old female with a bite wound.

Ms. Jones sits in a chair, filing her long, purple fingernails. Braids of black hair flow from atop her head down to her shoulders. She removes her dark glasses and gives you a cursory glance as you walk in the room. She pushes her glasses back in place and resumes work on her nails, all the while chomping and popping her chewing gum.

"Ms. Jones, what brings you in today?" you ask.

"A two-bit hussy bit me, that's what."

"Who or what bit you?"

"Tracy did, that's who."

"Who's Tracy?"

"Don't know her last name. She tried to steal away one of my customers last night. I got in her face and we got in a tussle is all."

"Where did she bite you?"

"Right here, on the arm." Ms. Jones points to her right upper arm.

"Any other injuries?"

"Nah, she only bit me once. I slapped her so hard on the side of the head she backed off."

Inspecting the patient's upper arm, you see two red arcs, like two tiny horseshoes, facing away from each other.

Looks like a bite wound, that's for sure.

"Did it break the skin? Did it bleed?"

"Some," replies the patient. "Look, I got to go, I just came in for a tetanus shot."

"How long has it been since you've had a tetanus shot?"

"About three years, I reckon."

You Are the ER Doc!

Question 1 — You should:

A) Tell the patient she doesn't need a tetanus shot.
B) Recommend an antibiotic shot.
C) Recommend antibiotics by mouth.
D) Scour the wound with rubbing alcohol until the patient cries for mercy.
E) Call the police to report the patient as a suspicious person.

Answer —

A) is correct.

"Tetanus shots are good for ten years for a wound like this, Ms. Jones. You don't need one."
"Think I need an antibiotic?"
"Antibiotics won't help prevent infection in this type of wound. If you develop infection in the wound later, that's another matter."
"Guess I be wastin' my time here, then. Don't need nothing."
"Maybe not. Let's talk about other possibilities."

Question 2 — You should:

A) Advise the patient about the risk of hepatitis.
B) Advise the patient about the risk of AIDS.
C) Advise the patient about the risk of local infection in the wound.
D) Ask whether the patient wants to file a police report.
E) All of the above.

Answer —

E) is correct. Any situation with possible transfer of body fluids (blood, urine, saliva, etc.) is complicated: In theory, potential for transmission of AIDS or hepatitis exists.

"Do you want to be checked for other infections? If the person who bit you had hepatitis or AIDS, it's possible you could get them from her."
"Say what?"

133

"There's a tiny chance you could get infected if the person who bit you is sick. Or, she could get sick from you if you're infected."

"She ain't sick, she's just a witch. And I had my test last month. I don't have it."

"You might not know if this Tracy person had the virus in her body. She might not look sick yet."

"How much chance I got, getting something from being bit?"

"As far as I know, there's only been once case of AIDS ever that was passed by a human bite. Your chances of getting AIDS are probably less than one in a million — less than the chance of getting AIDS just by having unprotected sex with a person."

"Reckon I already take that chance enough, then."

"Would you like us to test you for hepatitis and AIDS? We'd have to draw a blood test now and again in six weeks."

"Nah, I ain't got time for all that jazz."

"Would you like us to call the police so they can take a report?"

"No need to call the blue dogs. I already took care of Miss Tracy Witch myself."

"Suit yourself. The main thing you need to watch for is wound infection, since bite wounds are contaminated with lots of germs. Wash the wound every day, then put antibiotic ointment on it. If you see any signs of infection, come back right away."

"Yo, you can bet I'll be back lickety-split if I see any infection." ❖

Tricky Trauma

You are the emergency medicine doctor on duty in the Hometown Hospital Emergency Department.

"Hometown Hospital, this is Medic 4," the report comes from the radio.

"Hometown Emergency Department, go ahead Medic 4," Nurse Able says into the receiver.

"We're inbound with a 33 year-old female involved in a motor vehicle accident. Her car ran off the road into a ditch. The patient is awake but combative. Initial blood pressure 128 over 84. Pulse is up at 128. We had trouble getting her on a backboard and a putting a collar on her neck. She's flailing her arms and swearing, fighting everything we do, but she's finally immobilized now. Her skin is sweaty. She's got a one-inch cut on her scalp and a quarter-sized, red bruise on her forehead. We suspect internal head injury."

"Right, Medic-4. IV line established?"

"10-4, Hometown ED. Normal saline running at keep vein open. We'll be at your back door in five minutes."

The ambulance rolls to a stop, lights flashing. The medics promptly deliver your patient to Treatment Room 2, where you, two nurses and a technician stand waiting.

"OK, let's get her onto our stretcher," you say. "On three. One, two, three, lift."

Hands on all sides of the wooden backboard lift the patient from one stretcher to the other.

As you begin to examine your patient, her jaw clenches shut and her face turns beet red. Her arms and legs jerk spasmodically.

"Seizure," you say. "Able, grab some IV Valium to give if her seizure lasts more than a minute."

The jerking activity stops after 30 seconds. The young lady looks like she's asleep, but her skin is drenched with sweat. She begins to take long, deep breaths, restoring oxygen to her brain and muscles.

Question 1 — You should proceed at once with:
A) Asking the patient what happened.
B) A quick exam of the patient.
C) A finger-sensor check of the patient's oxygen level.
D) A finger-prick check of the patient's blood glucose (blood sugar).
E) A side view of the patient's neck vertebrae (cervical spine).
F) Notifying X-ray to have the CAT scan machine ready to get a CAT scan of the patient's brain.
G) All of the above.

Answer —

G) is correct. Get all the information you can.

"Ms. Rogers! Ms. Rogers, wake up!" you shout in the patient's ear.

The patient continues to take long, deep breaths, in and out. Her eyes remain closed, her arms and legs floppy-loose.

"Post-ictal, sleepy after the seizure," you say. "No way to get a history."

"Let's get vital signs, an oxygen saturation, and a fingerstick glucose. Get X-ray to shoot a stat, cross-table cervical spine film. And tell radiology to hold the CAT scanner open. We'll need a stat CT scan of the brain."

You begin to examine the patient again. Aside from the inch-long cut on her scalp and a bruise on her forehead, the patient has no sign of external injury to the head, chest, or abdomen.

"Blood pressure 148 over 88," Able reports. " Pulse 130. Respirations 16 per minute."

"Oxygen saturation is 100%," a technician adds.

"Blood glucose is low at 34."
"Whoa, hold the horses," you say.

Question 2 — You should:
  A) Get the neck X-ray done first.
  B) Send the patient for a CAT scan of the brain, since she has a cut scalp, bruised forehead, and is acting funny.
  C) Check a pregnancy test before doing any X-rays, since radiation could harm a developing fetus.
  D) Give a solution of concentrated sugar (D-50) intravenously.
  E) Re-examine the patient.

Answer —
  D) is correct.

"Let's give an amp of D-50, IV push, now!"
"D-50 going in," Able says. She shoves with her palm on the end of a large, glass syringe, pushing the contents into the patient's IV line.
The young lady opens her eyes.
"Where am I? What happened?" she says.
"Hometown Hospital," you answer.
"Are you a diabetic?"
"Yes, I take insulin."
"Your sugar got too low. You had a car wreck."
"Oh, my." She frowns. "I didn't hurt anyone, did I?"
"No. You drove off the road into a ditch. Nobody else was hurt. Speaking of which, do you have any pain anyplace? Does your head or neck hurt?"
"My forehead is a little sore, like I bumped it. Otherwise, I feel fine."
"OK, but I want you to hold still until I examine your neck and spine. If they're OK, we'll get you off this backboard."

Medical note: As in life, events in medicine are not always as they seem. In this case, hypoglycemia (low blood sugar) masqueraded as head trauma. ❖

You Are the ER Doc!

Get the Lead Out?

Your patient is: Danny Mills, a 41 year-old male who reports he's swallowed a pencil.

"Doc, I was sittin' there in McDonald's, drinkin' a cup of coffee, working a crossword puzzle. Had a pencil in my mouth, chewin' on the end of it, when some clown comes along and bumps my arm."

Mr. Mills pauses, peers down the end of his nose at the salt-and-pepper beard running from his chin to his belt buckle. With a flick of a long, thin, finger, he knocks a smattering of bread crumbs from the tangle of hairs.

He continues, "Next thing you know, I swallered the pencil right down. All the way into my stomach. Guess the grease from the french fries helped it along."

"Did you choke on the pencil?" you ask. "Any breathing difficulty then or since?"

"Naw, it slid right down the pike, smooth as silk. And my breathin's fine, it's the same as always."

Mr. Mills points a nicotine-stained finger at a faded, red gym bag on the floor. "Brought my bag along, too, doc, in case you need to put me in the hospital and maybe do surgery to get the pencil out."

Question 1 — You should:
  A) Examine Mr. Mills.
  B) Give Mr. Mills an antidote for lead poisoning immediately.
  C) Call a surgeon at once to operate and take the pencil out.
  D) Take an X-ray to look for the pencil inside Mr. Mills.
  E) Call McDonald's to confirm Mr. Mills's story.

Answer —

> A) is correct. Being a competent doctor, you examine your patient first.

"Let's take a look at you, Mr. Mills. Say, 'Aah'.
"Your throat is clear. No scrape or bleeding.
"Breathe deep, in and out.
"Your lungs have some coarse breath sounds. Hitting the cigarettes pretty heavy these days?"
"Two, sometimes three packs a day, doc."
"Terrible for you, Mr. Mills," you admonish. "Now lie down so I can examine your abdomen."
Pulling up Mr. Mills's shirt to examine his belly, your eyes widen. The pink skin on Mr. Mills's abdomen is criss-crossed by white, healed surgical scars.
"What surgeries have you had?" you ask, trying not to sound incredulous.
"Appendix, gall bladder, ruptured intestine, ulcers. You name it, I've had it."

> **Question 2** — You should:
>
> A) Give Mr. Mills an antidote for lead poisoning at once.
> B) Call a surgeon at once to take the pencil out.
> C) Take an X-ray to look for the pencil inside Mr. Mills.
> D) Call McDonald's to confirm Mr. Mills's story and order a couple Big Macs.
> E) Re-examine the patient.
>
> **Answer —**
>
> C) is correct. Find out if the pencil really is inside Mr. Mills. No antidote is necessary, since pencil lead is nontoxic graphite, not toxic lead.

Ten minutes later, the X-ray tech hands you a manila envelope. "Pencil, plus, I'd say," she says.
You pull the flimsy, celluloid sheets from the folder and snap them onto X-ray viewboxes on the wall. The fluorescent lights flicker to life behind the films. You stand back to peruse the X-rays.

You Are the ER Doc!

"Holy, tomole!" you say. Visible on the film are *two* faint, linear objects, capped by metal, and a *third* faint object about three inches long, topped by a metal cap and ring.

"Two pencils *and* a cigarette lighter," you say. "In the stomach."

Question 3 — You should:

A) Advise Mr. Mills to get treatment elsewhere since he is not telling you the whole truth and nothing but the truth.

B) Call social services to investigate a possible case of middle-age abuse.

C) Call a specialist to remove the objects by endoscopy (a lighted tube passed through the mouth into the stomach).

D) Call a psychiatrist to see Mr. Mills.

E) Ask the patient if he was somehow using two pencils and a cigarette lighter to work the crossword puzzle.

F) Both C) and D).

Answer —

F) is correct. Mr. Mills needs the objects removed from his stomach by endoscopy. The objects should be removed promptly, before they pass far into the intestine and have to be removed by surgery. Mr. Mills also needs psychiatric help, since it appears he suffers from a mental disorder causing him to swallow objects. He may even suffer from Munchhausen's syndrome. Patients with Munchhausen's syndrome go to extreme lengths to get into hospitals. They often cause harm to themselves or fake symptoms of conditions requiring surgery or other invasive procedures.

"Mr. Mills, you have more than a pencil in your stomach."
"What do we need to do, doc, surgery?"
"No, I'm calling an intestinal specialist to do an endoscopy. You've probably had that done before?"
"Lots of times, doc."
"I suspected as much. Have you seen a psychiatrist before, for your problem with swallowing things?"
Mr. Mills grins. "How'd you know that, doc?"
"Just a hunch, Mr. Mills. Just a hunch."

"I'll do whatever you say, doc. Just as long as you put me in the hospital and take good care of me."

"That we'll do, Mr. Mills." ❖

The Drip

Your patient is: Fenwick Stanton, a 20 year-old male.

The young man sits on the stretcher. He thumps a book shut as you walk in the room.

"Interesting reading?" you ask.

"Nah. Chemistry 101. We have final exams at the university this week."

"Well, good luck. But let's talk about what brings you to the emergency department. The chart says you're having trouble with your glands. What kind of trouble?"

"It's not my glands, doctor. That's just what I told them when I signed in out front. Actually, I've got a drip from my penis. I'm afraid I caught something at a fraternity party last weekend."

"Is it draining pus? White or yellow, and thick?"

"Yes, pus. It leaves a yellow stain in my underwear."

"Any fever, joint pain, sore throat, or skin rash?"

"No, just the drip. I'm fine, otherwise."

"No sores on your penis? No flu-like symptoms?"

"Nope."

"Let's have a look," you say, sitting down on a stool. "Stand up and slide your pants down."

The young man eases off the stretcher and stands in front of you. He unbuckles his belt and lets his blue pants and silk boxer shorts fall to his ankles.

With your gloved hand, you feel and look at all sides of Mr. Stanton's penis and testicles. No ulcers or lumps are present. The only abnormal finding is a drop of yellow pus oozing from the hole at the end of the penis.

Question 1 — You should:

A) Exclaim, "Oh, gross!" and tell the patient you don't treat sexually-transmitted diseases.
B) Warn the patient his penis may drop off.
C) Call the young man's parents to report his problem.
D) Take a swab of the pus and look at it under a microscope.
E) Treat the patient for pubic lice (crabs).

Answer —

D) is correct. You must know what Mr. Stanton has to treat him correctly.

"Mr. Stanton, you obviously have an infection in your penis. I'll make a microscope slide so we can identify which germ is causing the infection."

You dab at the pus on the tip of Mr. Stanton's penis with a long Q-tip. The yellow goop adheres to the white fibers on the swab. Rubbing the cotton on a microscope slide, you create a thin film of pus on the slide.

"This specimen goes to the lab for a gram stain. We should know what you have in about 30 minutes."

"Can I wait in the lobby, doctor?"

"Sure. I'll call you back and talk to you in private when the report on the smear comes back."

Forty minutes later, the ward secretary attaches the report to Mr. Stanton's chart and hands the chart to you.

The young man is studying his textbook again as you walk in the room.

"What's the verdict, doctor?" he asks.

"The slide showed you have gram-negative diplococci bacteria in the cells that line your penis. In simpler terms, you have gonorrhea."

"Gonorrhea?" The young man's eyes open wide. "For real?"

"No doubt about it."

"I can't believe I have gonorrhea." The young man shakes his head back and forth. "How do we get rid of it?"

YOU ARE THE ER DOC!

Question 2 — You should treat the patient with:
- A) One small shot.
- B) A single pill by mouth.
- C) Surgery to remove the affected part.
- D) Two large shots and three different antibiotics by mouth.
- E) Either A) or B).

Answer —
- E) is correct. Gonorrhea germs are usually sensitive to a small dose of antibiotic by mouth or shot.

"Mr. Stanton, we can treat you for gonorrhea with a single dose of medicine, by mouth or by shot. Which do you prefer?"
"Are you kidding? Give me the pill."
"I'll write you a prescription. Can you get it filled now?"
"I'm driving directly to the pharmacy from here."

Question 3 — You should also:
- A) Advise the patient to tell his sexual partner(s) that she/he/they likely have gonorrhea.
- B) Advise the patient to be checked to make sure he does not have syphilis.
- C) Advise the patient his behavior makes him at risk for AIDS, too.
- D) Report the patient's disease to the county health department.
- E) Treat the patient for chlamydia, another sexually-transmitted disease.
- F) All of the above.

Answer —
- F) is correct.

"Mr. Stanton, infectious disease experts recommend you take an additional antibiotic to treat possible chlamydia infection, too."
"I could have chlamydia?"
"Yes, indeed. You could also have incubating syphilis, genital

herpes, or AIDS, all of which are passed through unprotected sex, the same as gonorrhea."

"Gonorrhea's bad enough. I sure don't want to get those other things. Gonorrhea is curable, but AIDS isn't."

"To be safe, I recommend you make an appointment at the county health department this week. They can test you for syphilis and AIDS, and make sure your gonorrhea is cured. I have to report your case of gonorrhea to the Hometown County Health Department, anyway, so they can try to prevent the spread of this infection. That's the law in our state."

"I'll make the appointment."

"One final piece of advice. I suggest you be more careful in the future. Either keep it in your pants or use a condom."

"You can bet I will, doctor. You can bet I will." ❖

You Are the ER Doc!

The Pregnancy Pukes

Your patient is: Melissa Carsdale, a 19 year-old female complaining of vomiting.

"Ms. Carsdale?"

"What's left of me," she answers.

The young lady lies on the stretcher, the back of her hand resting on her forehead. She opens her eyes and turns her head to face you.

"I just can't stop throwing up," she says. Dark circles surround her eyes, contrasting with her pasty face.

"Are you having fever or diarrhea?"

"No, just vomiting."

"Pain in your abdomen?"

"No."

"Any possibility you're pregnant?"

"I think so. I did a home pregnancy test and it was borderline positive. My period is three weeks late."

Ms. Carsdale grabs a pink emesis basin at her side, props herself up on one elbow, and retches into the basin. She heaves, and heaves again, shuddering with effort. Saliva and yellow liquid spurt in drivels from her mouth into the basin.

> **Question 1** — You should:
> A) Examine Ms. Carsdale.
> B) Order a urine pregnancy test.
> C) Do a urinalysis.
> D) Get an IV line going to give Ms. Carsdale IV fluids.
> E) All of the above are reasonable.
>
> **Answer** —
> E) is correct. You can examine your patient, make a diagnosis and treat, all at the same time.

Sticking your head out the door of the treatment room, you hail one of the nurses.

"Worthy, would you send a urine pregnancy test on Room 8? And a urinalysis?"

"Already sent," comes the answer.

"How about an IV line?"

"Name your flavor."

"Ringers lactate, at 500 cc's per hour."

Turning your attention back to Ms. Carsdale, you place your palm on her forehead. Tendrils of brown hair stick to the sides of her pallid face. Her skin is clammy.

"Open your mouth wide," you say.

Strands of mucus connect from Ms. Carsdale's tongue to the top of her mouth.

"How long have you been throwing up?"

"A whole week off and on, but worse the past two days," she says.

"You're dehydrated. The mucus membranes inside the mouth should be moist and shiny. The inside of your mouth is dry and sticky."

With your fingers, you push on all areas of Ms. Carsdale's abdomen. "Anyplace hurt when I press?" you ask.

"No hurting. It just gives me a queasy feeling."

Nurse Worthy enters the room, IV tubing and bag in hand. "The pregnancy test is positive," he says. "The urinalysis shows ketones and the specific gravity is 1.030."

You explain, "What Mr. Worthy means is that your urine is concentrated, and you're breaking down stores of body fat for food."

"And, also, we know what's making you throw up."

"What?" queries Ms. Carsdale.

Question 2 — You should tell the patient:

  A) Morning sickness.

  B) Morning, noon, and night sickness.

  C) The pregnancy pukes.

  D) Pregnancy-associated vomiting.

  E) Hyperemesis gravidarum.

  F) Any of the above.

Answer —
F) is correct.

"Ms. Carsdale, you have a bad case of morning sickness, which, in your case, is closer to 24-hours-a-day sickness. That's how it is with some unlucky mothers-to-be. It's miserable, especially for the first three months of pregnancy."

"Three months?" she gasps.

"Possibly," you answer. "Sometimes not that long. Sometimes longer than three months. But, today, we'll get you feeling better with some IV fluid. Just correcting your dehydration with fluid by vein will perk you up, and also buy some time until you can keep liquids down by mouth."

"Will all this vomiting hurt me? And what about the baby? Will it harm the baby?"

Question 3 — You should tell the patient:

A) She may suffer kidney damage but the baby will not be harmed.

B) She will be fine, but the baby is more likely to have birth defects.

C) The baby might be born with a camel-like hump so it can store water.

D) People that have bad morning sickness usually have twins, triplets, or even quadruplets.

E) She may be uncomfortable, but the baby will be fine.

Answer —
E) is correct.

"You may feel miserable, Ms. Carsdale, but we're going to make sure you suffer no harm. The only danger is dehydration, a lack of fluids inside your body, since you can't keep down liquids by mouth. We're going to correct your dehydration today and then get an OB doctor to provide follow-up treatment.

"As for the baby, he or she will suffer no harm. Your baby will get what it needs from you. Babies born to mothers with pregnancy-associated vomiting do not suffer harm or birth defects. If anything, they tend to do a little better than babies born to mothers who don't have morning sickness."

"That makes me feel better."

"I thought it might."

"But what causes this problem?"

"Nobody knows, at least not yet."

"What about medicine to stop the vomiting?"

Question 4 — You should:

A) Tell Ms. Carsdale not to worry. You will give her some medicine now by vein and prescribe some suppositories.

B) Carefully discuss with Ms. Carsdale the use of medicines in pregnancy.

C) Tell Ms. Carsdale federal law prohibits the use of any medicine except vitamins in pregnant females.

D) Advise Ms. Carsdale you can't prescribe medicine, but there is medicine available at health food stores she can take.

E) Advise Ms. Carsdale the FDA (Food and Drug Administration) won't approve it, but there is a medicine called NoVomik which is available through mail order from Mexico.

Answer —

B) is correct.

"Any medicine should be used during pregnancy only if necessary. We should consider the risks and benefits, just like in non-pregnant patients. Only now we need to consider the well-being of two patients, you *and* the baby. We have to be extra careful if a medicine is given in early pregnancy, while the baby is developing, because the medicine could cause birth defects."

"Should I take anything for the vomiting, then?"

"That's a decision you must make. We have medicine that can help control the vomiting, and it is pretty safe in pregnancy. The medicine has been given to lots of mothers without any obvious pattern of birth defects in their babies. But the possibility of a medicine harming the baby always exists."

"I'll have to think about it. I may need to take the medicine. I just can't stand feeling like this all the time."

"That's fine. We'll use the safest medication we can if you decide you want a prescription."

You turn to walk out of the room. Ms. Carsdale's clothes, piled on a chair next to the stretcher, catch your eyes. A pack of cigarettes protrudes from her shirt pocket.

Question 5 — You should:

A) Snatch the cigarettes out of her shirt pocket, shout "Down with the evil tobacco weed," and crush the pack under your shoe.

B) Ignore the cigarettes, as it's none of your business.

C) Call the police: Ms. Carsdale is too young to smoke.

D) Call Ms. Carsdale's parents to see if they are aware she has been smoking.

E) Warn Ms. Carsdale about the hazards of smoking during pregnancy.

Answer —

E) is correct. Perhaps the most important action you take today is to get Ms. Carsdale to stop smoking.

"Ms. Carsdale, there is another very important change you need to make for your baby's sake."

"What is that, doctor?"

"You absolutely, positively, must stop smoking. You have your own health to consider, and now the health of your baby. Smoking is harmful to your baby's development. Smoking causes lower birth weight and birth defects."

"I won't touch another cigarette, I promise."

"I hope so, both for your sake and for the sake of your baby. And, remember, after the baby's born, even secondhand smoke is harmful. Please don't take up smoking again, for your child's sake."

"I'm giving up cigarettes for good, doctor."

"That would be an excellent gift to give yourself and your family-to-be, young lady." ❖

Snakebit

You are the emergency medicine doctor on duty in the Hometown Hospital Emergency Department.

"I got bit, I got bit!" yells the man bursting through the double doors of the emergency department.

Close on the man's heels is a beefy security guard. "I couldn't stop him, doc," says the guard, huffing and puffing. "His friend's got the snake that bit him in a jar."

"Let me get you into a room," says Nurse Able to your new patient. She grabs the long-haired, dirt-stained, white t-shirt and blue-jean clad man by the arm, and leads him toward a treatment room. "Got a name?" she says.

"Jimmy. Jimmy Tiller," he says. "Don't let me die, please don't let me die. The gol-durn snake bit me," he adds, obediently following Nurse Able.

"You'll be OK, Mr. Tiller," Nurse Able says, automatically reassuring.

Realizing the potential for a true emergency, you stride into Room 4 right behind the pair.

Nurse Able yanks the blue curtain in the front of the room shut. "Let's get your shirt off, Mr. Tiller," she says, helping the patient lift his t-shirt over his head.

She raises the back of the stretcher. "Sit up here," she says.

Mr. Tiller sits on the stretcher. He is breathing at twice the normal rate.

Quicker than you can ask, Nurse Able wraps a blood pressure cuff around the patient's arm. "168 over 98," she says seconds later.

"How do you feel right now, Mr. Tiller?" you ask.

"My heart's a-poundin'. Feel like I'm a'goin' to die," he says.
"Almost did coming here, too. My buddy drove as fast as his pickup would go, and we 'bout got in two wrecks on the way here."
"Where did the snake bite you?"
"Here on the arm." The patient fingers a dirt-smudged area on the top of his forearm.

No swelling, bruising, or bleeding show where he points. Small, pinpoint, red dots, in the shape of a V, are faintly visible.

Question 1 — You should:
    A) Tie a tight tourniquet on the arm above the dots.
    B) Apply cold to the bitten area.
    C) Cut the skin dot-to-dot with a scalpel, then tell the patient to apply suction with his mouth.
    D) Administer snake antivenin.
    E) Leave the patient and go check the snake.

Answer —
    E) is correct.

"Mr. Tiller, I'm going to go take a look at the snake," you say. "I believe you're going to be OK."
"Ain't you going to cut it, doc, to get the poison out? Do it if you got to, I can take it."
"Cutting your arm or tying a tourniquet on, or even putting a cold pack on, can do more harm than good for a poisonous snake bite. Let me go see if the snake looks poisonous before we do anything."
"He's got diamond markings on his back, doc. I know he's a poison 'un!"
"Let me see what his other markings show first, Mr. Tiller."
You easily locate Mr. Tiller's friend in the waiting room – he sits in a seat with a gallon-sized pickle jar on his lap. No one sits in the seats on either side of him.
"Let's take a look at this critter," you say. Mr. Tiller's friend hands you the jar without a word.
You lift the hefty jar with both hands and hold the glass in

front of your nose. The serpent within flicks a black tongue in and out of its mouth.

"Is it poisonous?" says Nurse Able.

"No way, Jose," you answer. "See the round pupils? Poisonous snakes have slit pupils, just like cats. And there's no pit between the nose and the eye, and the head's not sharply triangular.* No, this is a corn snake — not dangerous, unless you're a mouse."

"So why is the patient hurting? His breathing is fast and his blood pressure is up, too."

"He's scared. The man thinks he's been bitten by a poisonous snake, so he's hyper and the adrenaline is pumping. He'll calm down when I tell him he's going to be fine."

Your reassuring hand goes on Mr. Tiller's shoulder. "You're going to be A-OK, captain. The snake is not poisonous."

"You sure, doc?"

"Sure as if I got bit myself. You need a tetanus shot and the wound cleaned, then you'll be ready to go."

Nice job, doctor. Way to sift through the facts. No use getting excited over nothing. ❖

---

* Medical note: The coral snake is the only poisonous snake in the United States without slit pupils, a heat-sensing pit, and a triangular head. A coral snake has round pupils, no pit, and a round head. The coral snake has distinctive red, yellow and black bands circling the length of its body. Other snakes have similar markings. Just remember, if the red and yellow bands touch each other, "Red and yellow can kill a fellow." Fortunately, coral snake bites are very rare.

Snakebite

Your patient is: Danny Rivers, a 12 year-old boy bitten by a snake.

"You'll feel a stick," Nurse Able says. She hovers over the boy's arm, a small, shiny needle in hand, intent upon the task of starting an IV line.

Danny manages a half-grimace, half-smile. White teeth contrast with his tanned face. His mop of brown hair is highlighted with a natural, sun-bleached layer on top.

"How'd you get bitten?" you ask the boy. "And when?"

"About a half hour ago," he answers. "I threw my bike down next to a ditch. When I was getting back on the bike, I felt a sting on my ankle. I looked down and saw a snake in the weeds."

"What did the snake look like?"

"Brown, about two feet long, not very big. It shook its tail and buzzed a little, but it wasn't the regular rattlesnake sound like you see on *Wild America* and shows like that."

"What happened then?"

"My ankle felt like it was on fire. I yelled for my Dad, and he drove me here in his truck."

"Let's take a look at your ankles."

Danny pulls up the legs of his blue sweat pants. The left ankle is noticeably larger than the right. Two tiny puncture wounds, a half-inch apart, stare like eyes in the middle of a three-inch-bruise face, located just above the bone on the outside of the ankle.

The boy's left calf is larger than his right calf. Swelling reaches all the way up to the knee.

You Are the ER Doc!

Question 1 — Danny has sure signs of:
  A) Faking an injury to get attention.
  B) A bite from a rabid (infected with rabies) animal.
  C) A snakeweed sting, which mimics a snakebite.
  D) A bite from a snake — either poisonous or nonpoisonous.
  E) A bite from a snake — a poisonous one.

Answer —
  E) is correct.

"Danny, there's no doubt you were bitten by a poisonous snake. You've got two fang marks, pain, bruising, and swelling. I'm afraid it got you, kid."

The boy nods. "I figured that was the case." He raises his eyebrows and asks, "Do you have to cut the fang marks with a knife?"

Question 2 — Your next step is to:
  A) Immediately cut an X over the marks with your pocket-knife, then tell the boy to suck the wounds with his mouth.
  B) Cut the fang marks with a sterile scalpel, then apply suction with a machine.
  C) Tie a tight tourniquet on the leg above the swelling.
  D) Apply cold to the bitten area.
  E) Prepare to administer snake antivenin.

Answer —
  E) is correct. The most important treatment of a poisonous snakebite (a serious case) is antivenin.

"Danny, we won't cut you, I promise. Cutting and sucking doesn't do any good. If somebody sucks on a wound with his mouth, it may create a worse problem because mouth germs get in the wound and cause infection."

The boy smiles. "I'm glad you don't have to cut me."

"We do need to get some antivenin in your veins to counteract the poison. Quickly. Do you understand, compadre?"

Danny nods. "Will it hurt?"

"We'll draw some blood for tests, and I have to prick you with two small needles to make sure you're not allergic to the antivenin. The needle sticks hurt a bit, but they've got to be done. OK?"

"I can take it," he answers.

Your hand goes on the boy's shoulder.

"You're a good patient, Danny, a lot better than even most adults would be. That helps us a lot. I'm going to get your dad back here to explain what we're doing and tell him how brave you are."

"Can he stay back here with me?"

"You bet."

You're on the ball, doctor. No hesitation on this one: Aggressive and specific treatment is necessary to save the boy's leg and perhaps even his life. ❖

INDEX

alcoholic 37, 98, 115
appendicitis 121

baby, delivery of 113
BB gun injury 78
bean in the nose 79
bee sting 20
bite wound, animal 47
bite wound, human 132
bladder, foreign body 83
bleach, ingestion 33
bug in the ear 37

chest pain 85

drip 142

ectopic pregnancy 13

fever 27, 58, 61
fever, infant 61
fox lick 48

gonorrhea 143

hand infection 55
heroin overdose 9
hip fracture 129
HMO 88

intubation 104, 122

Jehovah's Witnesses 16

laceration, arm and chest 125
laceration, face 66
lead pencil, ingestion 139
living will 25, 106

maggots 40
meningitis 30
millipede 99
Munchhausen's syndrome 140

pregnancy, ectopic 13
pregnancy, unexpected 111
pregnancy-associated vomiting 148

rabies 46, 49
religious refusal 31
reptiles 70
roach 39

Salmonella bacteria 70
seizure 72, 136
shingles 51
snakebite, nonpoisonous 152
snakebite, poisonous 155
squirrel bite 45
stroke 22, 103, 106
subdural hematoma 117
suitcase sign 43, 138

taillight sign 42
tetanus booster 46

ABOUT THE AUTHOR

Peter Meyer, MD, lives with his family in Wilmington, North Carolina.

Dr. Meyer graduated from Miami (Ohio) University with a Bachelor of Arts degree in zoology. He was elected to Phi Beta Kappa.

In 1978, Dr. Meyer received his Doctor of Medicine degree from the Ohio State University. He was elected to Alpha Omega Alpha.

Subsequently, Dr. Meyer completed a residency in internal medicine at the Bowman-Gray School of Medicine in Winston-Salem, North Carolina.

For the next 18 years, Meyer practiced emergency medicine in Wilmington, North Carolina. He became board-certified in emergency medicine in 1986, and he remains so to date.

Dr. Meyer is a successful writer and publisher. Other books by Dr. Meyer include:

- *Nature Guide to the Carolina Coast: Common Birds, Crabs, Shells, Fish, and other Entities of the Coastal Environment* (a widely-acclaimed book about the environment and common plants and animals of the Carolina coast)

- *Blue Crabs: Catch 'em, Cook 'em, Eat 'em* (a practical and comprehensive guide to blue crabs, crabbing, and blue crab cookery on the Atlantic and Gulf Coasts)

- *Medicalese: A Humorous Medical Dictionary* (a tongue-in-cheek look at medicine and medical terminology)

The author is pictured on the front cover of this book.

You Are the ER Doc!

can be ordered by mail.

Books ordered by mail are shipped promptly.

Every book ordered by mail is signed by the author.

Books can be personalized, too.
Print (legibly) the name(s) of the person(s) to whom the book is to be signed.

(for example, "to Bob and Sally")

Order form

Send a check or money order only.

Name _____

Address _____

City _____ State _____ Zip _____

Send _____ copies of *You Are the ER Doc!* at $11.95 _____

Shipping for the first book $1.50 _____

Shipping for each additional book $ .50 _____

NC residents add tax per copy of $ .72 _____

TOTAL _____

Personalize to:

Make checks payable to **AVIAN-CETACEAN PRESS**.
Mail order to:
Avian-Cetacean Press, PO Box 15643, Wilmington, NC 28408